ECG Companion For Beginning Experts

Electrocardiography (ECG) has existed in the medical field for over 100 years, but important concepts are still beyond the horizon for some trainees and physicians alike. This book occupies an unfilled niche, written for physicians, trainees and advanced practitioners across various specialties. Using a case-based format, it provides an analytical system that facilitates a high-yield interpretation, and by breaking down the 12-lead ECG using a simple system, the learner can quickly identify important findings. Thus, it serves as a practical tool to strengthen the knowledge of health care providers and facilitate better understanding and management of patients with abnormal ECGs—regardless of their career paths through the medical field.

Key Features:

- Utilizes a two-pronged explanation style to facilitate learning where the first prong is the "what" of the ECG, and the second prong is the "why" and "how."
- Focuses on high-yield abnormalities and clinical pearls to enable those providers outside of the cardiology space to become more knowledgeable and confident when interpreting ECGs.
- Uses a built-in question bank to test and reinforce concepts learned in the primer and case studies.

ECG Companion For Beginning Experts

On Chen, MD

Associate Authors

Ryan F. Heslin, MD MBA

Jahan Manjur, MD

Abhijeet Singh, MD

Mark Jacobs, MD

Andreas Kalogeropoulos, MD PhD MPH

CRC Press

Taylor & Francis Group

Boca Raton London New York

CRC Press is an imprint of the

Taylor & Francis Group, an **informa** business

Designed cover image: www.shutterstock.com/image-photo/heart-wave-red-line-beat-isolated

First edition published 2025
by CRC Press
2385 NW Executive Center Drive, Suite 320, Boca Raton FL 33431

and by CRC Press
4 Park Square, Milton Park, Abingdon, Oxon, OX14 4RN

CRC Press is an imprint of Taylor & Francis Group, LLC

ISBN: 978-1-032-93321-4 (hbk)
ISBN: 978-1-032-93319-1 (pbk)
ISBN: 978-1-003-56538-3 (ebk)

DOI: 10.1201/9781003565383

Typeset in Times
by KnowledgeWorks Global Ltd.

Dedicated to Ioana, my love, my rock, and my inspiration. And to Nhomi, Adam, and Noam—my three rays of light who illuminate my path. To Zlila, Amnon and Toot, for the unconditional love and unwavering support. This work is as much yours as it is mine.

~ On Chen

ASSOCIATE AUTHORS

To my beautiful wife and wonderful children—thank you for making me a better person
To Chad, Matt, Mike, Paul, and Ravi—thank you for being the best co-fellows I could've asked for
To Hal, Noelle, Robert, and On—thank you for being amazing mentors for every step of my journey!

~ Ryan F. Heslin

I would like to dedicate this book to my wife, Ghazal, for her unwavering support throughout this journey, and to my wonderful children, Zaina and Aariv, for their boundless joy and inspiration.
I also extend my gratitude to my parents for their enduring encouragement and love.

~ Abhijeet Singh

Dedicated to my grandfather, William Schwartz, who instilled in me the notion that one of the noblest causes is to share knowledge through teaching, and to my parents, grandparents, sisters, and friends; without their support, I could not have accomplished so much.

~ Mark Jacobs

To Hal Skopicki, a brilliant physician and more importantly an extraordinary person. Your steadfast dedication to your team, your genuine investment in our professional growth and deep care of our personal well-being have inspired us beyond measure. This book is testament to values you instill in all of us: compassion, commitment, and excellence.

~ Ryan F. Heslin, Jahan Manjur, Mark Jacobs, Abhijeet Singh, Andreas Kalogeropoulos, and On Chen

Contents

Preface

The purpose of this primer is to provide a foundation of knowledge for the internal medicine resident in efficient and accurate interpretation of electrocardiograms (ECG) in the setting of various cardiovascular diseases and potentially life-threatening conditions. The American Board of Internal Medicine (ABIM) deems appropriate ECG testing and interpretation of results as a required clinical competency. Despite this requirement, recent literature highlights the need for improvement in ECG interpretation among residents of internal medicine.

The content found in this primer aims to guide the reader in a systematic evaluation of the ECG and more specifically prepare residents for the ABIM—Internal Medicine Boards (which contains 14% in the cardiovascular disease section, the largest section of subject matter by percentage). All illustrations contained within this primer are either the original artworks of the authors or protected under creative commons (and have been credited with authorship) where applicable. All ECGs contained within this primer have been de-identified to protect the identity of our patients. Special thanks to our patients who provide us with valuable teaching material every day.

Below are some notable resources to aid in the above endeavor:

- Electronic Resources
  - Dr. Smith's ECG Blog (http://hqmeded-ecg.blogspot.com)
  - EMergugate Blog (http://www.emergucate.com)
  - Dr. Ken Grauer Blog (http://ecg-interpretation.blogspot.com)
  - Life in the Fast Lane (https://litfl.com/)
  - ECG Pedia (https://en.ecgpedia.org/)
  - ECG Wave Maven (https://ecg.bidmc.harvard.edu/maven/mavenmain.asp)
  - "ABC of Clinical Electrocardiography" Series (BMJ)—See PubMed
- Book Resources
  - *The Only EKG Book You'll Ever Need* by Malcolm Thaler MD
  - *The Complete Guide to ECGs* by James H. O'Keefe Jr. MD et al.
- Reference Textbooks
  - *Marriott's Practical Electrocardiography* by Galen S. Wagner
  - *Hurst's The Heart* by Valentin Fuster MD

About the Author

Dr. On Chen, MD, FACC, FSCAI, is an interventional cardiologist and the director of the cardiac intensive care unit and the telemetry units at Stony Brook University Hospital (SBUH). He is the founding director of the Cardiogenic Shock Program; he also serves as the director of outpatient cardiology services and the Advanced Lipid Management Program. Dr. Chen has published numerous research studies and serves as the principal investigator in several multi-center trials. He has dedicated his career to educating students, residents, and fellows. He has authored multiple curricula for various cardiology rotations offered at SBUH and is spearheading quality improvement projects to improve resident and fellow well-being while also contributing to high-value patient care.

Associate Authors

Dr. Ryan F. Heslin, MD MBA, received his undergraduate degree from Stony Brook University, his MBA from Stony Brook University College of Business, and his MD from Stony Brook Medical School. He was inducted into the Alpha Omega Alpha (AOA) Honor Society and won the Excellence in Basic Science Research award for his research on burn injury progression and in vitro angiogenesis. Dr. Heslin completed internal medicine residency at Stony Brook University Hospital (SBUH) and is currently a fellow in the Stony Brook Cardiology Fellowship. He has also authored numerous publications in internal medicine and cardiology, taken part in cardiology clinical trials, and is interested in cardiology education. Dr. Heslin is privileged to begin working as a noninvasive/imaging attending physician at SBUH in 2025.

Dr. Jahan Manjur, MD, is a graduate of Stony Brook University. He subsequently obtained his medical degree at St. George's University. He completed his residency at Stony Brook University Hospital (SBUH) and completed fellowships in Cardiovascular Diseases and Interventional Cardiology at NY Presbyterian—Brooklyn Methodist Hospital. During residency training, he took particular interest in ECG interpretation and helped start the ECG Club at SBUH for the Internal Medicine residents. Currently, he is in practice as an interventional cardiologist serving North Jersey as a faculty member at Englewood Health Medical Center (EHMC). He continues to be passionate about ECGs and helps teach ECG interpretation to the house staff at EHMC.

Dr. Abhijeet Singh, MD, is an assistant professor of medicine at SUNY-Stony Brook University, New York. Serving as associate program director of the cardiology fellowship program, he has a keen interest in the education of medical students, residents, and fellows. Apart from conducting regular ECG lectures and "Transition to Residency" series for medical students, he plays an active role in the electrophysiology lecture series for cardiology fellows. Practicing as a cardiac electrophysiologist and being able to perform and interpret intracardiac electrograms and device interrogations gives him a keen insight into subtleties of surface ECGs. This book is an attempt to reduce the anxiety associated with ECGs for all levels of trainees.

Dr. Mark Jacobs, MD, received his BS from University of Miami and his medical degree from the Albert Einstein College of Medicine, where he achieved distinction in clinical research. He completed a residency in internal medicine at the University of Miami/Jackson Memorial Hospital program, where he went on to serve as a chief resident in quality and safety at the Bruce W. Carter Veterans Affairs Hospital in Miami, Florida. He then went on to complete fellowships in cardiovascular disease at Stony Brook University Hospital (SBUH) and advanced heart failure and transplant cardiology at New York Presbyterian—Weill Cornell Medical Center. He is currently a fellow in critical care medicine at Montefiore Medical Center while also completing an executive MBA/MS program in healthcare leadership at Cornell. He is passionate about cardiovascular clinical research, quality improvement, and medical education.

Dr. Andreas Kalogeropoulos, MD, MPH, PhD, FACC, FHFSA, FASE, is associate professor of medicine and the director of cardiovascular research at Stony Brook University, Long Island, New York. He is a clinical researcher with expertise in heart failure, echocardiography, and research methodology. Dr. Kalogeropoulos graduated from the University of Patras, Greece (MD, 1994), where he completed his training in internal and cardiovascular medicine (2004) and research methodology (PhD, 2012). He joined Emory University, Atlanta, GA, in 2006, where he trained in echocardiography, heart failure, and outcomes research (MPH, 2013). Dr. Kalogeropoulos has authored over 200 peer-reviewed articles and 5 book chapters, and he is the lead editor in a major heart failure textbook. His research focuses on (1) risk factors, outcomes, and clinical prediction models for patients with heart failure or at risk for heart failure, with the goal to optimize management; and (2) applications of cloud computing using large electronic health records networks for outcomes research and regulatory applications in cardiovascular disease.

Overview

On Chen

This primer will roughly follow the ACC/AHA list of diagnoses on the previous page as the method of classification. It should be noted that not all topics will be discussed explicitly. The references provided at the beginning of this text are available (HSC Library and VAMC Library) to fill any gaps in knowledge.

BASIC STRATEGY*

The following is a commonly used strategy in the evaluation of an ECG.

Rate and Regularity

- Heart rate (atrial and ventricular, if pertinent)
- Regularity (atrial and ventricular, if pertinent)

Rhythm Analysis

- Basic Rhythm (sinus, ectopic, atrial or ventricular)
- Ectopic or intermittent rhythms (PACs/PVCs)

Waveforms of the ECG

- P-wave morphology and origin (axis, enlargement)
- PR interval (short, normal, or long)
- QRS width (narrow or wide)
- QT interval (correction, if needed)
- Presence of pathological Q-waves
- ST-segment analysis (elevations, depressions, reciprocal changes)
- T-waves (morphology, inversions)
- QRS axis (deviations)
- Presence of U-waves

* There are many strategies for ECG evaluation. Whichever method is used, it is important to stay consistent to guarantee a thorough and complete assessment of the ECG.

Conduction Analysis

- Any conduction blocks (sinoatrial, atrioventricular, etc.)
- Any intraventricular blocks (bundle branch, fascicular, and nonspecific blocks)

Final ECG Interpretation

- Conclusion and overall impression

ELECTROCARDIOGRAPHIC DIAGNOSES

Below is a list of ECG diagnoses from the 2001 ACC/AHA Clinical Competence Statement on Electrocardiography and Ambulatory Electrocardiography:

NORMAL TRACING

- ❑ Normal ECG

TECHNICAL PROBLEMS

- ❑ Leads misplaced
- ❑ Artifact

SINUS NODE RHYTHMS AND ARRHYTHMIAS

- ❑ Sinus rhythm
- ❑ Sinus tachycardia
- ❑ Sinus bradycardia
- ❑ Sinus arrhythmia
- ❑ Sinus arrest or pause
- ❑ Sino-atrial exit block

OTHER SUPRAVENTRICULAR RHYTHMS

- ❑ Atrial premature complexes
- ❑ Atrial premature complexes, non-conducted
- ❑ Ectopic atrial rhythm
- ❑ Ectopic atrial tachycardia, unifocal
- ❑ Ectopic atrial tachycardia, multifocal
- ❑ Atrial fibrillation
- ❑ Atrial flutter
- ❑ Junctional premature complexes
- ❑ Junctional escape complexes or rhythm
- ❑ Accelerated junctional rhythm
- ❑ Junctional tachycardia, paroxysmal

VENTRICULAR ARRHYTHMIAS

- ❑ Ventricular premature complexes
- ❑ Ventricular escape complexes or rhythm
- ❑ Accelerated idioventricular rhythm
- ❑ Ventricular tachycardia
- ❑ Ventricular tachycardia, polymorphous
- ❑ Ventricular fibrillation

ATRIAL VENTRICULAR CONDUCTION

- ❑ First-degree AV block
- ❑ Mobitz Type I second-degree AV block (Wenckebach)
- ❑ Mobitz Type 2 second-degree AV block
- ❑ AV block or conduction ratio, 2:1
- ❑ AV block, varying conduction ratio
- ❑ AV block, advanced (high-grade)
- ❑ AV block, complete (third-degree)
- ❑ AV dissociation

INTRAVENTRICULAR CONDUCTION

- ❑ Left bundle branch block (fixed or intermittent)
- ❑ Right bundle branch block (fixed or intermittent, complete or incomplete)
- ❑ Intraventricular conduction delay, nonspecific
- ❑ Aberrant conduction of supraventricular beats
- ❑ Left anterior fascicular block
- ❑ Left posterior fascicular block
- ❑ Ventricular pre-excitation (Wolff-Parkinson-White pattern)

QRS AXIS AND VOLTAGE

- ❑ Right axis deviation (+90 to +180 degrees)
- ❑ Left axis deviation (−30 to −90 degrees)
- ❑ Indeterminate axis
- ❑ Electrical alternans
- ❑ Low voltage

CHAMBER HYPERTROPHY OR ENLARGEMENT

- ❑ Left atrial enlargement, abnormality, or conduction defect
- ❑ Right atrial abnormality
- ❑ Left ventricular hypertrophy (QRS abnormality only)
- ❑ Left ventricular hypertrophy with secondary ST-T abnormality
- ❑ Right ventricular hypertrophy with or without secondary ST-T abnormality

REPOLARIZATION (ST-T,U) ABNORMALITIES

- ❑ Early repolarization (normal variant)
- ❑ Juvenile T waves (normal variant)
- ❑ Nonspecific abnormality, ST segment and/or T wave
- ❑ ST and/or T wave suggests ischemia
- ❑ ST suggests injury
- ❑ ST suggests ventricular aneurysm
- ❑ Q-T interval prolonged
- ❑ Prominent U waves

MYOCARDIAL INFARCTION

- ❑ Inferior MI (acute or recent)
- ❑ Inferior MI (old or age indeterminate)
- ❑ Posterior MI (acute or recent)
- ❑ Posterior MI (old or age indeterminate)
- ❑ Septal MI (acute or recent)
- ❑ Anterior MI (acute or recent)
- ❑ Anterior MI (old or age indeterminate)
- ❑ Lateral MI (acute or recent)
- ❑ Lateral MI (old or age indeterminate)
- ❑ Right ventricular infarction (acute)

CLINICAL DISORDERS

- ❑ Chronic pulmonary disease pattern
- ❑ Acute pericarditis
- ❑ Suggests hypokalemia
- ❑ Suggests hyperkalemia
- ❑ Suggests hypocalcemia
- ❑ Suggests hypercalcemia
- ❑ Suggests CNS disease

PACEMAKER

- ❑ Atrial-paced rhythm
- ❑ Ventricular-paced rhythm
- ❑ Atrial-sensed ventricular-paced rhythm
- ❑ AV dual-paced rhythm
- ❑ Failure of appropriate capture, atrial
- ❑ Failure of appropriate capture, ventricular
- ❑ Failure of appropriate inhibition, atrial
- ❑ Failure of appropriate inhibition, ventricular
- ❑ Failure of appropriate pacemaker firing
- ❑ Retrograde atrial activation
- ❑ Pacemaker mediated tachycardia

FIGURE 0.1

Source: Kadish, A. H., Buxton, A. E., Kennedy, H. L., Knight, B. P., Mason, J. W., Schuger, C. D., Tracy, C. M., Winters, W. L., Boone, A. W., Elnicki, M., Hirshfeld, J. W., Lorell, B. H., Rodgers, G. P., Tracy, C. M., & Weitz, H. H. (2001a). ACC/AHA clinical competence statement on electrocardiography and ambulatory electrocardiography. *Circulation*, *104*(25), 3169–3178. https://doi.org/10.1161/circ.104.25.3169)

The Normal ECG, and Introduction to Sinus Rhythm

1

Ryan F. Heslin and Jahan Manjur

THE NORMAL ECG

	P wave	QRS complex	T wave	U wave
Duration	80–110 ms	60–100 ms	–	–
Axis	0° to 75°	−30° to +105°	–	–
Morphology	I, II: upright *aVF*: upright or inverted III, *aVL*, V_1, V_2: inverted or biphasic	–	I, V_3–V_6: upright *aVR*, V_1: inverted III, *aVL*, *aVF*, V_2: upright, flat, or biphasic	Upright except aVR
Amplitude	*Limb*: <2.5 mm V_1: (+) <1.5 mm (−) <1 mm	–	*Limb Leads*: <6 mm *Precordial Leads*: <10 mm	5%–25% of T wave height (usually <1.5 mm)
Notes	Small notching may be present in the P wave, may be normal	*Transition Zone*: V_2–V_4 *Q Wave*: (<40 ms, <2 mm) common in aVR, V_1, V_2	*Juvenile T wave*: TWI in V_1–V_3 may be present in healthy young adults	–

FIGURE 1.1

DOI: 10.1201/9781003565383-1

	PR interval	ST segment	QT interval
Duration	120–200 ms	–	300–440 ms (corrected)
Notes	PR segment usually isoelectric Considered elevation >0.5 mm and depression >0.8 mm	Usually isoelectric Limb leads may vary <1 mm V_2–V_3 (V_4) up to 3 mm concave upward elevation in young adults, usually <2 mm in age 40+	*Bazett's Formula*: $QT_c = \frac{QT}{\sqrt{RR}}$

FIGURE 1.2

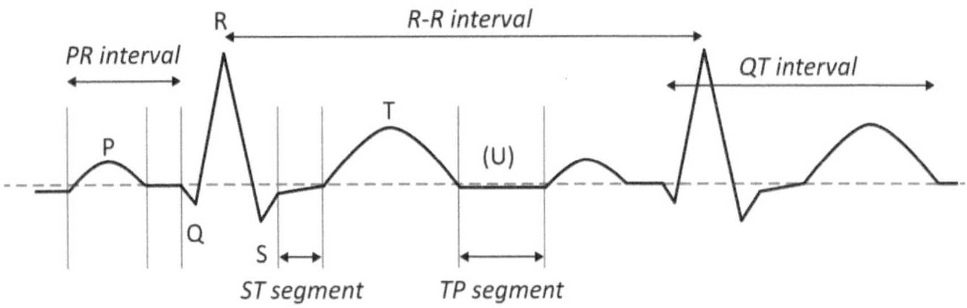

FIGURE 1.3

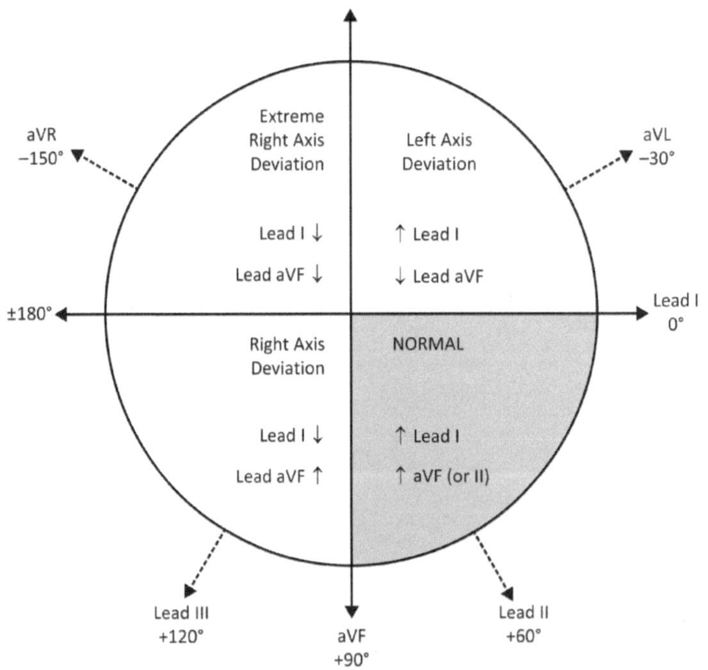

FIGURE 1.4

Naming the QRS complex

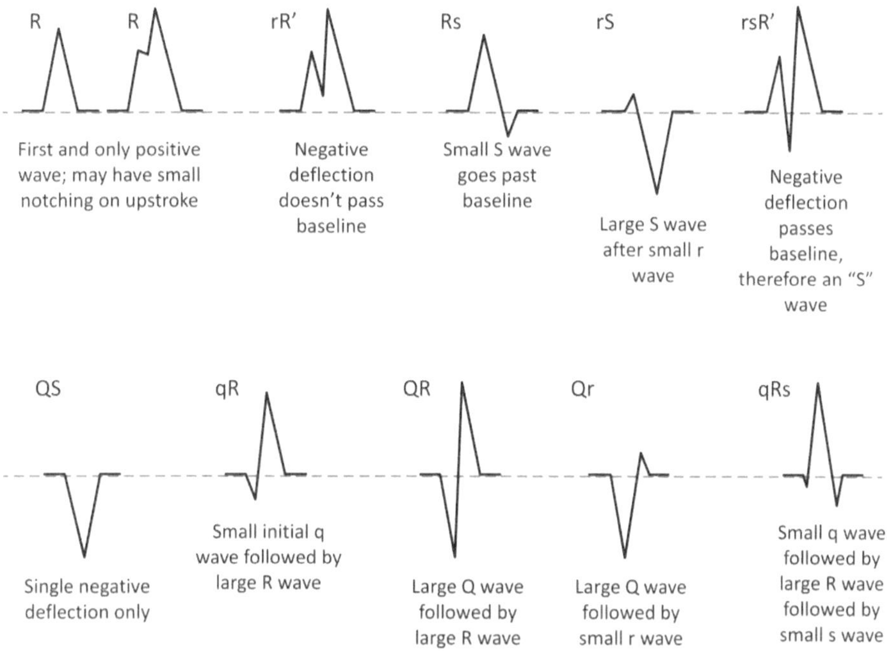

FIGURE 1.5

P WAVE AND ATRIAL ENLARGEMENT

The P wave

- Represents atrial depolarization, sequentially from the R to L atria
- *Abnormalities* best seen in inferior leads and V_1
  - P. Pulmonale (seen in RAE)
  - P. Mitrale (seen in LAE)
  - Inversions [↓] = ectopic or junctional rhythms

Bi-atrial enlargement

- Criteria of LAE and RAE present on same ECG
  - Listed below

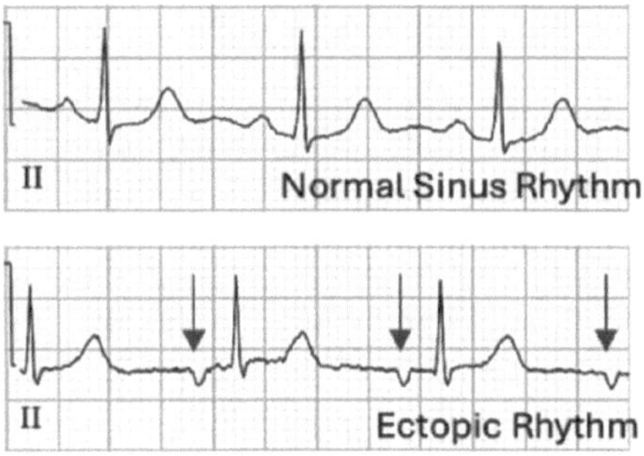

FIGURE 1.6

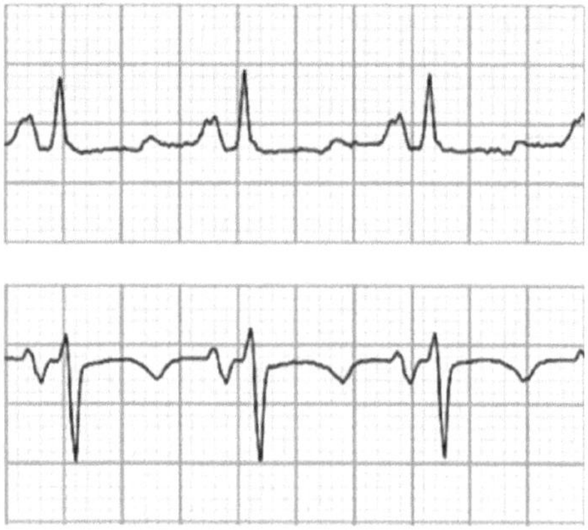

FIGURE 1.7

Left atrial enlargement (either)

- Terminal (-) P-wave in V_1 (>1 mm and 40 ms)
- Notched P-wave >120 ms in the inferior leads
    - P. Mitrale classically due to mitral stenosis

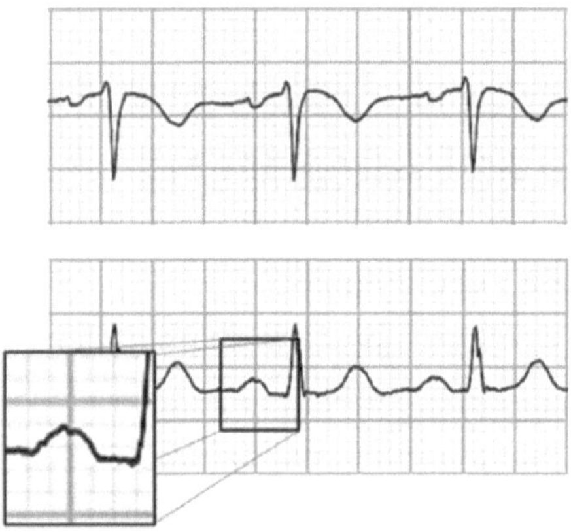

FIGURE 1.8

Right atrial enlargement

- Tall upright P-waves (either)
    - 1.5 mm in V_1, V_2
    - >2.5 mm in II, III, aVF (P. pulmonale)

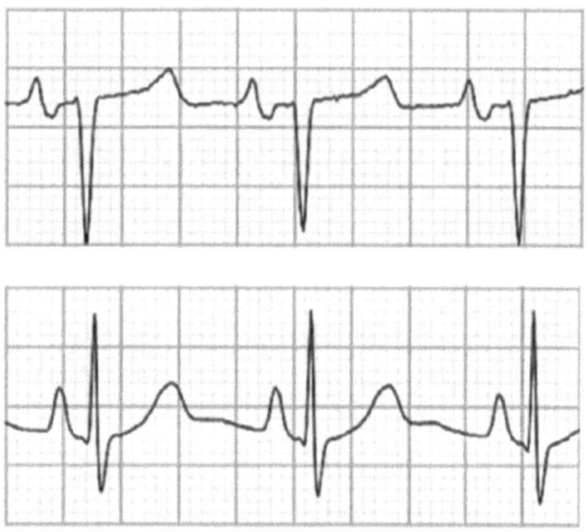

FIGURE 1.9

SINUS RHYTHMS AND ARRHYTHMIAS

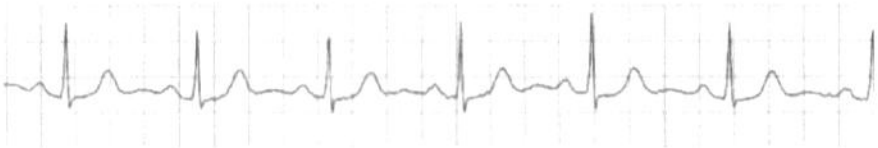

FIGURE 1.10

Normal Sinus Rhythm

- Normal P-wave axis and morphology
- Atrial rate of 60–100 BPM
- Regular (PP variance <160 ms or <10%)

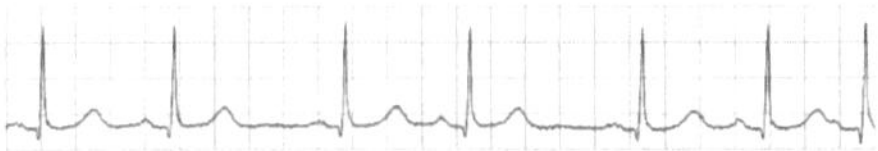

FIGURE 1.11

Sinus Arrhythmia

- Normal P-wave axis and morphology
- Respirophasic variance to PP interval
- PP variance >160 ms or >10%

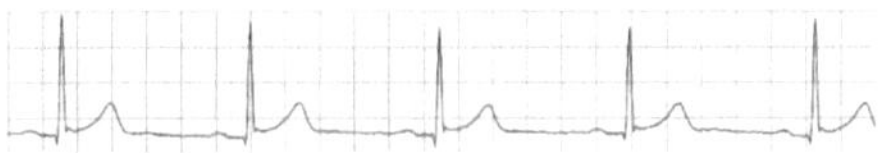

FIGURE 1.12

Sinus Bradycardia

- Normal P-wave axis and morphology
- Atrial rate of <60 BPM

NB: If rate of <40 BPM, consider 2:1 block

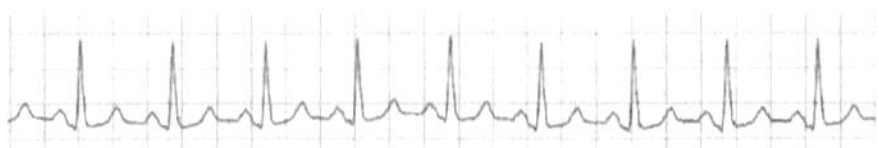

FIGURE 1.13

Sinus Tachycardia

- Normal P-wave axis and morphology
- Atrial rate of >100 BPM

NB: P amplitude may increase; PR may decrease

Sinus Pause or Arrest

- PP interval >1.6–2.0 seconds
- **<u>Not</u> a multiple of basic sinus PP interval**

Sinoatrial Exit (SA) Block

NOT the same as AV Block which has identical classification; ONLY second-degree sinoatrial block diagnosable on surface ECG

First-degree

- Delay between SA node impulse and atrial depolarization; cannot be seen on a surface ECG

Second-degree

- P wave morphology consistent with sinus rhythm
  - **Type I (Mobitz I/ Wenckebach) Sinoatrial Exit Block**
    - Progressive lengthening of the SA node impulse to atrial depolarization (but in decreasing length of delay) leading finally to transmission failure
    - "Group beating"
      - (1) Shortening of PP interval up to pause
      - (2) Constant PR interval
      - (3) PP pause <2× the normal PP interval

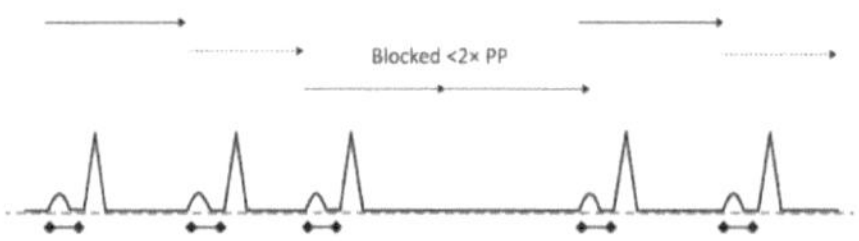

FIGURE 1.14

  - **Type II (Mobitz II) Sinoatrial Exit Block**
    - Constant PP interval followed by a pause that is a multiple (e.g., 2×, 3×, etc.) of normal PP interval
    - The pause may be slightly less than twice the normal PP interval (usually within 100 ms)

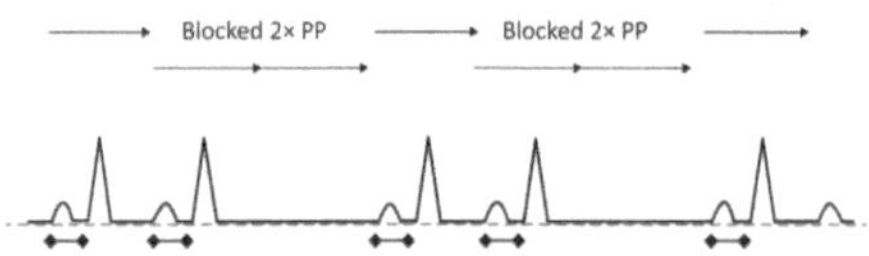

FIGURE 1.15

Third-degree

- Complete failure of sinoatrial conduction; cannot be differentiated from complete sinus arrest on a surface ECG

BIBLIOGRAPHY

1. O'Keefe, J. H., Pogwizd, S. M., Freed, M. S., & Hammill, S. C. (2015). *The ECG Criteria Book* (2nd ed.). Jones & Bartlett Learning.

Atrioventricular and Intraventricular Conduction Abnormalities

2

Ryan F. Heslin and Jahan Manjur

AV CONDUCTION ABNORMALITIES

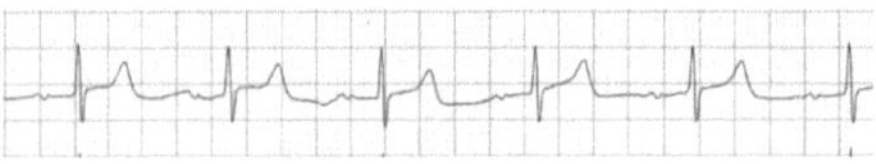

FIGURE 2.1

1° AV Block (1° AV Delay)

- PR interval >200 ms (up to 800 ms):
  - *Not representative of SA node to atrial conduction, but interval between atrial and ventricular depolarizations*
  - Narrow QRS, if site of block is near the AV node
  - Wide QRS indicates delay in the His-Purkinje system
- Each P-wave is followed by a QRS complex

DOI: 10.1201/9781003565383-2

2° AV Block (Mobitz Type I/Wenckebach)

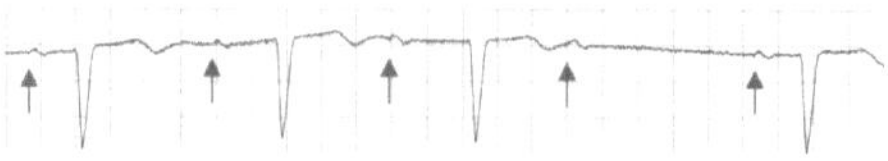

FIGURE 2.2

- PR prolongation, shortening R-R until dropped beat
- R-R containing non-conducted P-wave <2× the P-P
- PR intervals before & after dropped beat:
  - Non-constant PR intervals suggest Type I block
  - Constant PR interval suggests Type II block

NB: "Group" or "pattern beating" is not exclusive to Type I AVB

2° AV Block (Mobitz Type II)

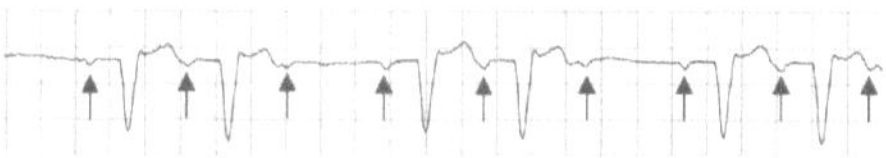

FIGURE 2.3

- Sinus or atrial rhythm with intermittent non-conducted P-waves without atrial prematurity
- PR interval in the conducted beats is constant
  - R-R with non-conducted P-wave exactly 2× the P-P

NB: 2:1 AVB can be Type I or II; exercise will not affect PR in Type II. NB: Type II AVB usually within or below the bundle of His; wide QRS 80%

3° AV Block

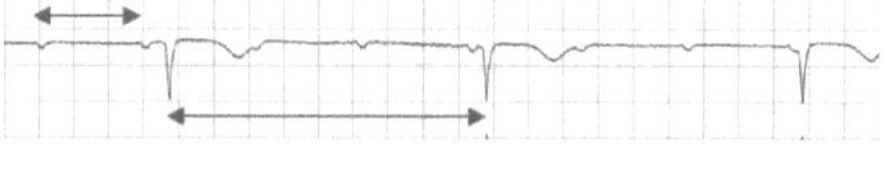

FIGURE 2.4

- Complete heart block where atrial impulses *consistently* fail to reach the ventricles (even when NON-refractory), leading to independent rhythms
- PR interval varies, *but* PP and RR intervals constant
- Atrial rate > Ventricular rate
  - P-waves may precede, be buried, or follow QRS

  - Ventricular rhythm maintained by a junctional or idioventricular escape rhythm
- Ventriculo-phasic sinus arrhythmia: P-P interval containing QRS complex shorter than PP interval without QRS

A-V dissociation (AVD): Independent atrial and ventricular rhythms without implying AVB, but both can occur concurrently as well

  - A secondary phenomenon to other dysrhythmias
  - **AVD without CHB: Only some atrial rhythms conducted (changing QRS morphologies)**

Isorhythmic AVD is when atrial and ventricular rhythms are nearly of equal rate and appear to be synchronized (rare)

Wolf-Parkinson-White Pattern

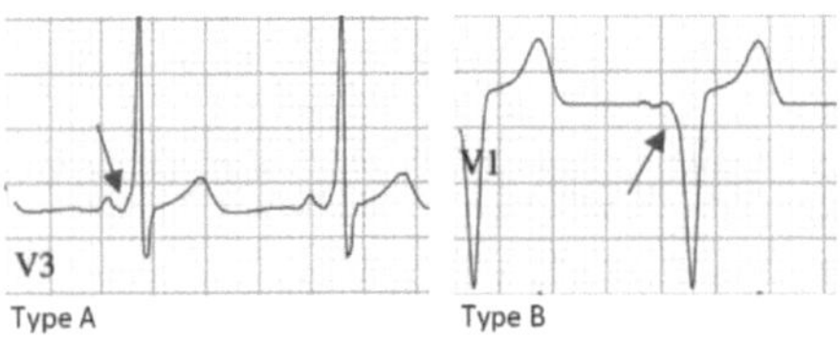

FIGURE 2.5

- ECG with a normal P-wave morphology and axis, but usually with a short PR interval (<120 ms)
- AV conduction via Bundle of Kent (accessory pathway) bypasses the AVN, thus pre-excitation of the ventricles
- With initial slurring of the QRS (delta wave), a wide QRS (>120 ms) represents fusion between the accessory pathway (delta wave ↓) and the AV node
- PJ interval remains constant, with an inverse relationship of PR interval and QRS duration
  - PR interval shortens, the QRS widens (vice versa)

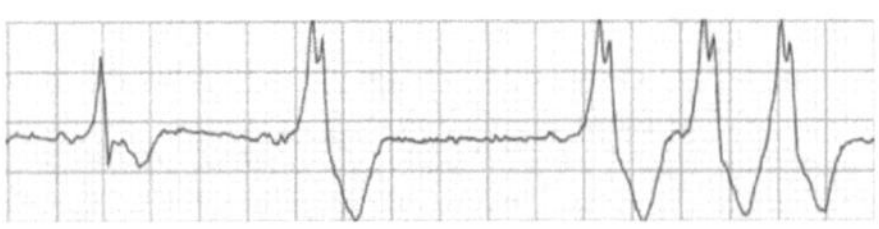

FIGURE 2.6

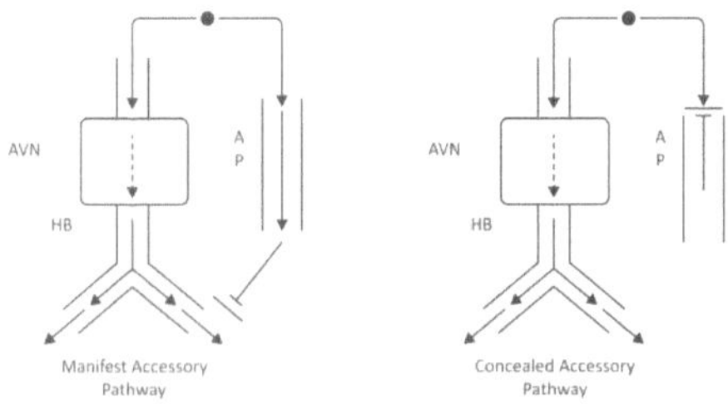

FIGURE 2.7

NB: Think WPW when AF/flutter with variable width QRS (generally wide) and rate >200 BPM

NB: AF can conduct extremely rapidly, leading to an irregular WCT (resembling VT) which can degenerate into VF

Wolf–Parkinson–White Syndrome

- Characterized by abnormal network of conduction tissue connecting the atrium and ventricle bypassing conduction through the AV node
- Two types of accessory pathways (AP) exist:
  - In manifest AP, antegrade conduction over the AP results in pre-excitation on baseline ECG (may be intermittent)
  - In concealed AP, antegrade conduction via the AV node and retrograde conduction occurs over the AP, so pre-excitation is not evident on baseline ECG
- Fifty percent of patients manifest tachyarrhythmias:
  - AVRT (80%), AF (15%), flutter (5%)
- Asymptomatic individuals have an excellent prognosis
- In patients with recurrent tachyarrhythmias, the overall prognosis is good (SCD is rare)
- Presence of delta waves and secondary repolarization abnormalities can lead to a false positive or false negative diagnosis of hypertrophy, BBB, or MI

INTRAVENTRICULAR CONDUCTION ABNORMALITIES

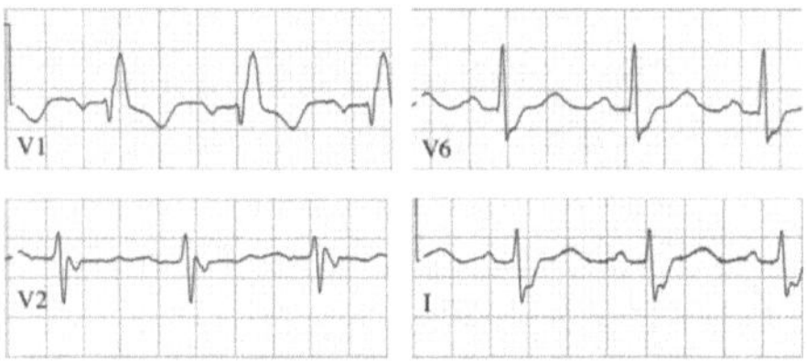

FIGURE 2.8

Complete Right Bundle Branch Block (RBBB)

- Prolonged QRS duration (>120 ms)
- Secondary R-wave (R') in leads V_1 and V_2 (rsR' or rSR') with R' wider than the initial R-wave
- Secondary ST-T changes (TWI; downsloping ST segment) in leads V_1 and V_2
- Wide (>40 ms) slurred S-wave in leads I and V_6
- If a dominant R-wave in lead V_1: delayed onset (>50 ms) of peak of R-wave, but normal in V_5–V_6

NB: Mean axis (determined by initial 60–80 ms of QRS), expected to be normal unless LAFB/LPFB is also present

NB: RBBB doesn't interfere with the ECG diagnosis of RVH/LVH or MI

NB: Seen in general population (no prognostic significance)

Incomplete Right Bundle Branch Block

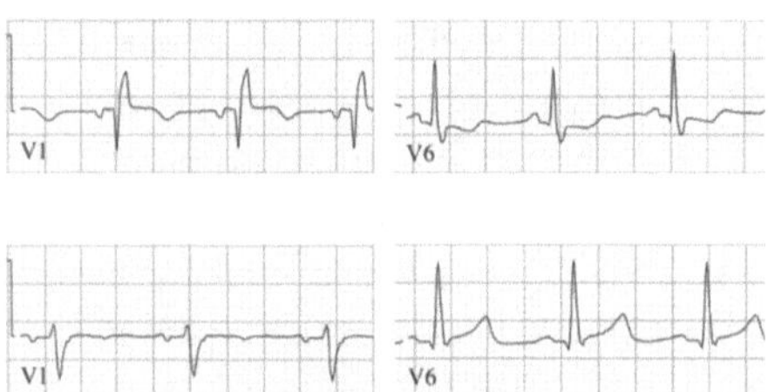

FIGURE 2.9

- RBBB morphology with QRS duration 110–120 ms
- Other causes of RSR' pattern <120 ms in lead V_1:
  - Normal variant, RVH, PWMI, lead placement, skeletal deformities, ASD

Non-specific Intraventricular Conduction Delay

- QRS of >110 ms, but doesn't meet full criteria for LBBB or

RBBB Nonspecific IVCD seen with LVH, WPW, antiarrhythmics, metabolic disturbances

Functional (Rate-Related) Aberrant Intraventricular Conduction

- Wide (>120 ms) QRS rhythm due to underlying SVT (including atrial fibrillation/flutter)

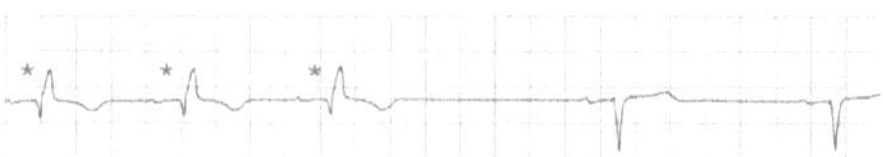

FIGURE 2.10

NB: Right bundle has a longer refractory period, thus aberrant conduction usually occurs down the left bundle, resulting in RBBB morphology

NB: Return to normal conduction may lead to T-wave abnormalities

Left Anterior Fascicular Block

- Left axis deviation between –45° and –90°
- qR complex (or an R-wave) in leads I and aVL
- rS complex in lead III
- Normal or slightly prolonged QRS (80–100 ms)
- Poor R wave progression is common

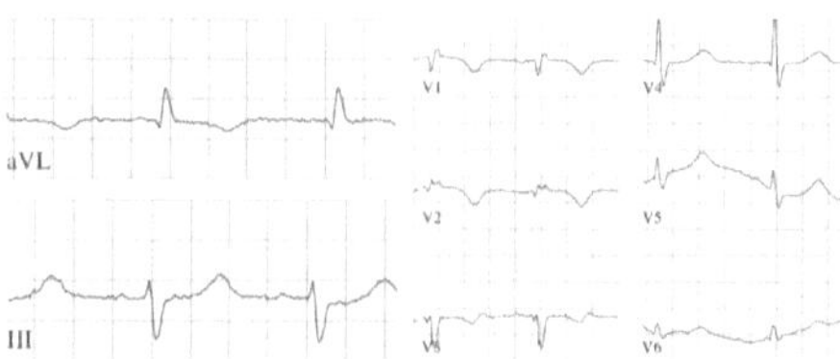

FIGURE 2.11

NB: LAFB can *mask the presence of inferior wall MI*

Left Posterior Fascicular Block

- Right axis deviation between +100° and +180°
- Normal or slightly prolonged QRS (80–100 ms)
- rS pattern in leads I and aVL
- qR pattern in leads III and aVF

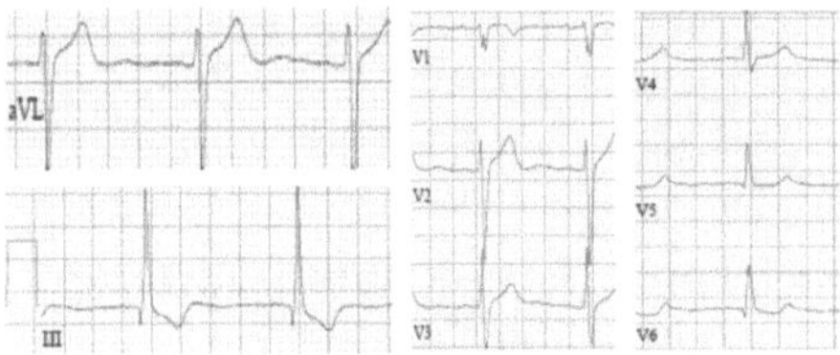

FIGURE 2.12

NB: LPFB can *mask the presence of lateral wall MI*

NB: LPFB is less prevalent due to dual blood supply; when it develops during acute MI, multivessel coronary disease and extensive infarction are usually present, with poor prognosis.

Complete Left Bundle Branch Block

- Prolonged QRS duration (>120 ms)
- Broad monophasic R-waves in leads I, aVL, V_5, V_6 usually notched/slurred (without q waves)
- Delayed onset (>60 ms) to peak of R-wave in leads V_5, V_6 but normal in V_{1-3} (if present)
- Secondary ST-T changes opposite in direction to the major QRS deflection
- ± Concordant T-waves, when positive QRS

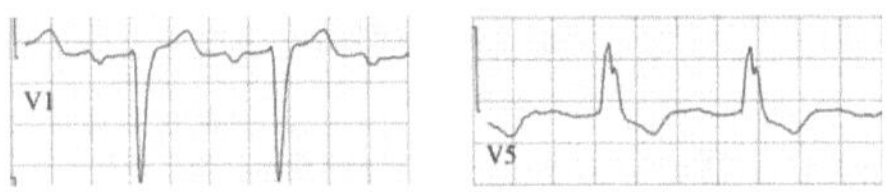

FIGURE 2.13

Incomplete Left Bundle Branch Block

- LBBB morphology with a QRS 110–120 ms
- Presence of LVH pattern
- R peak time greater than 60 ms in leads V_{4-6}
- Absence of q-wave in leads I, V_5, and V_6

BIBLIOGRAPHY

1. O'Keefe, J. H., Pogwizd, S. M., Freed, M. S., & Hammill, S. C. (2015). *The ECG Criteria Book* (2nd ed.). Jones & Bartlett Learning.

QRS Complex and Repolarization Abnormalities

3

Ryan F. Heslin and Jahan Manjur

QRS ABNORMALITIES

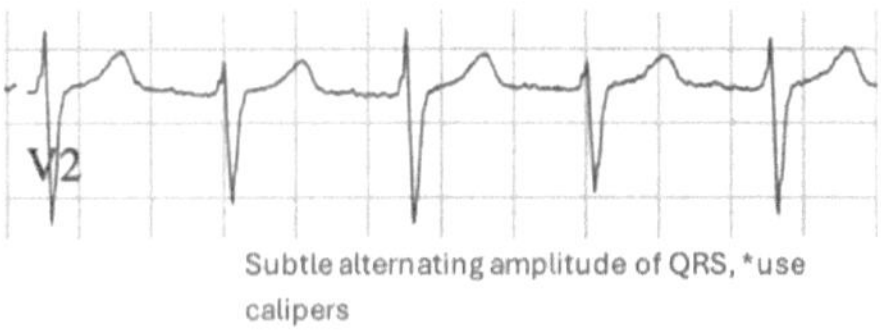

FIGURE 3.1

Electric Alternans

- Alternating amplitude and/or direction of the P, QRS, or T-waves
- Only 33% of patients with alternans have an effusion
- "Total alternans" (P-QRS-T), likely tamponade

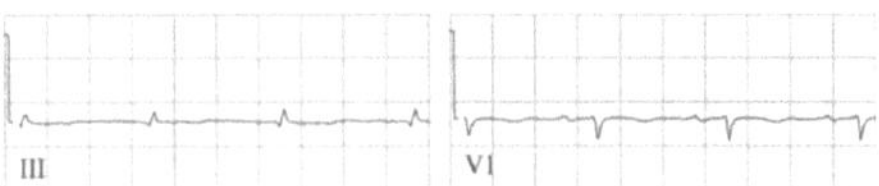

FIGURE 3.2

Low Voltage

- QRS (R+S) <10 mm in all precordial leads
- QRS (R+S) < 5 mm in all limb leads

DOI: 10.1201/9781003565383-3

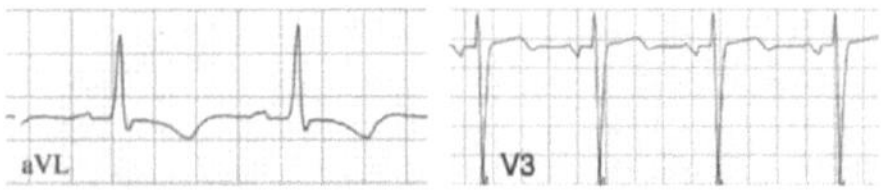

FIGURE 3.3

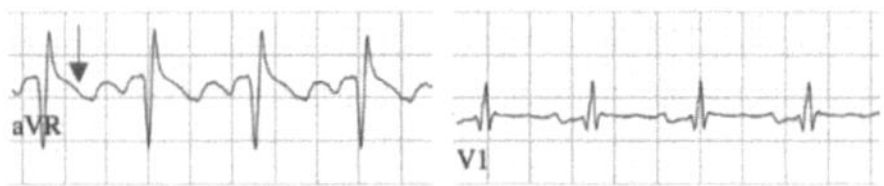

FIGURE 3.4

Left Ventricular Hypertrophy

Voltage criteria (sufficient without repolarization abnormalities)

- Cornell Criteria (most accurate, common)
  - R-wave in aVL + S wave in V_3
  - >28 mm in males or >20 mm in females
  - Other Criteria (Sokolow–Lyon, Romhilt–Estes)

Right Ventricular Hypertrophy

- Diagnostic yield of ECG diagnosis is low
- Right axis deviation with mean QRS axis $\geq +100°$
- Predominantly tall R-waves (part of Rs, R, or qR)
- Secondary ST-T changes [↓] (downsloping ST depression, TWI) notable in V_1 or aVR
- R/S ratio in $V_1 > 1$

Combined Ventricular Hypertrophy

Suggested by any of the following:

- ECG meets >1 criteria for LVH and RVH
- Precordial leads show LVH, but QRS axis is >90°
- LVH plus:
  - R>Q in aVR, S>R in V_5, and TWI in V_1
- Large amplitude, equiphasic R = S in V_3 and V_4 (Kutz–Wachtel phenomenon)
- Right atrial abnormality/enlargement with LVH pattern in precordial leads

REPOLARIZATION ABNORMALITIES

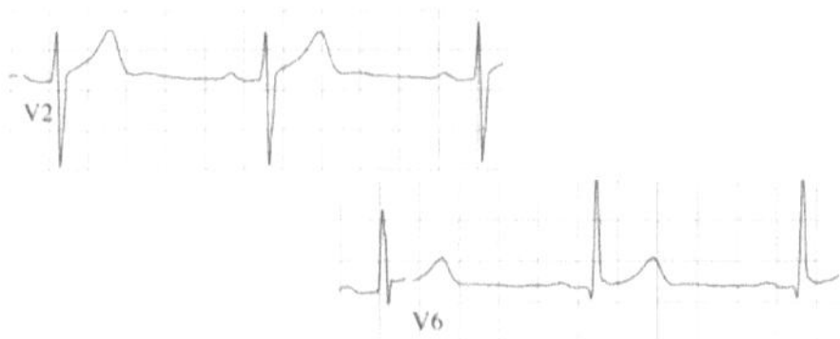

FIGURE 3.5

Normal Variant, Early Repolarization

- Elevated J (junction) point without reciprocal ST depressions
- Concave upward STE (<25% of T-wave in V_6) with a symmetrical upright T-wave
- Distinct notch or slur on downstroke of R-wave
- Most commonly involves V_2–V_5; sometimes in the inferior leads

Normal Variant, Juvenile T Waves

- Persistently negative T-waves (asymmetrical and shallow) in V_1–V_3
- T-waves still upright I, II, V_5, V_6
- More common in women and children, extremely rare in adult men

Prolonged QT Interval

*HR is crucial in QT correction as demonstrated by these examples to the right (NB: scale difference)

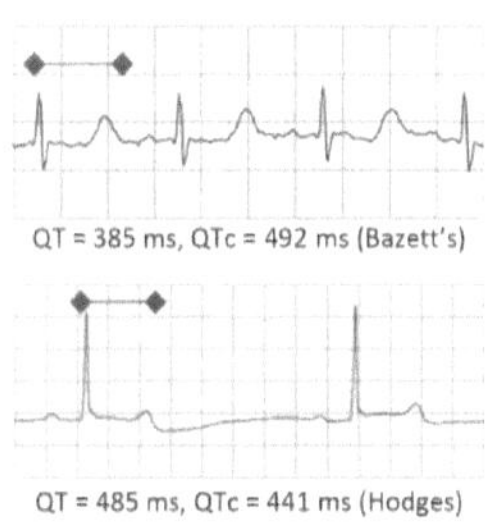

FIGURE 3.6

- QTc ≥440–460 ms (depending on gender)
- Easiest method to determine QT interval:
  - Generally, the normal QT interval should be <50% of the RR interval
- QT interval represents the period of ventricular electrical systole (i.e., ventricular depolarization and repolarization), varies inversely with HR, and is longer while asleep (due to vagal hypertonia)

- Many etiologies of QT prolongation (medications, electrolytes, congenital, etc.)
- Increased risk of ventricular arrhythmias

Prominent U-Wave

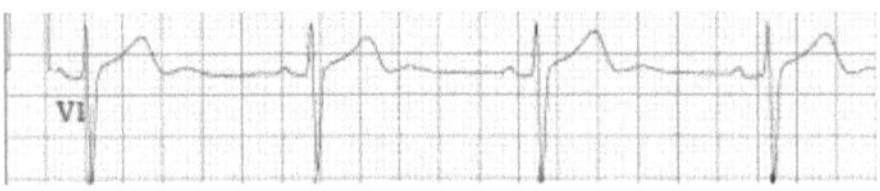

FIGURE 3.7

- Amplitude >1.5 mm, ~5–25% of the T-wave
- U-wave is normally largest in V_2, V_3

Nonspecific ST and/or T-Wave Abnormalities

- Slight (<1 mm) ST depression or elevation, and/or flat/inverted T-wave
- Seen in many conditions, highly non-specific

ST and/or T-Wave Abnormalities Suggesting Ischemia

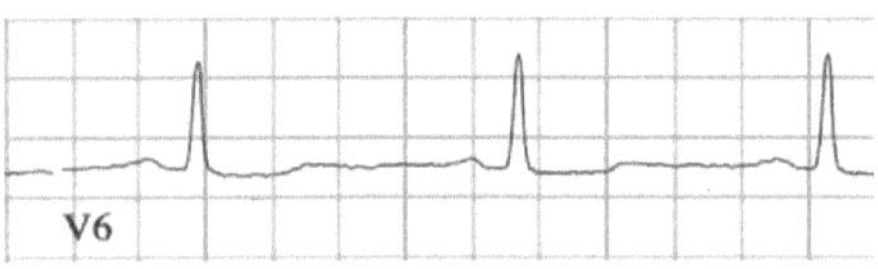

FIGURE 3.8

- *Ischemic ST changes*: Horizontal or downsloping ST segments ± T-wave inversions
- *Ischemic T-wave changes*: Biphasic T-waves ± ST depression; symmetrical or deep TWI; QT often prolonged
  - Reciprocal T-wave changes may be seen, or pseudo-normalization may occur
- Prominent U-waves (upright or inverted) may be present

ST and/or T-Wave Abnormalities Suggesting Injury

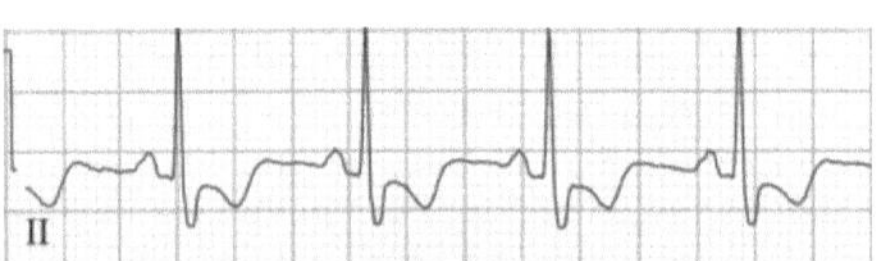

FIGURE 3.9

- Acute STE of <1 mm with upward convexity
- *ST and T-wave evolution*: T-waves invert before ST segments return to baseline

- Associated ST depression in the non-infarct leads
- Acute posterior wall injury often has horizontal or downsloping ST depressions with upright T-waves in V_1 and/or V_2 with prominent R-waves

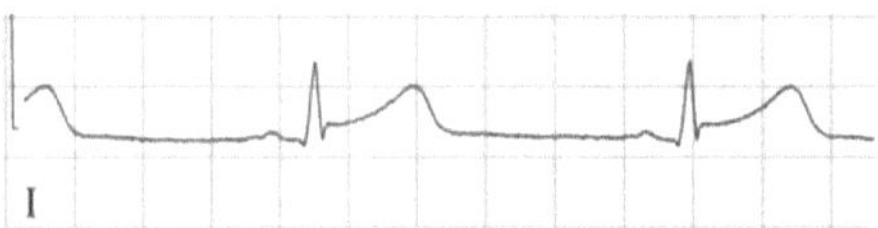

FIGURE 3.10

ST and/or T Abnormalities Secondary to Hypertrophy

- *LVH*: ST and T displacement opposite the QRS deflection:
  - STD (upwardly concave) and TWI when the QRS is positive (leads I, V_5, V_6)
  - Subtle (< 1 mm) STE and upright T-waves when the QRS is negative (leads V_1, V_2)
  - More extreme voltages, STE up to 2–3 mm can be seen in V_1–V_2
- *RVH*: ST depression and TWI in leads V_1–V_3 and sometimes leads II, III, aVF

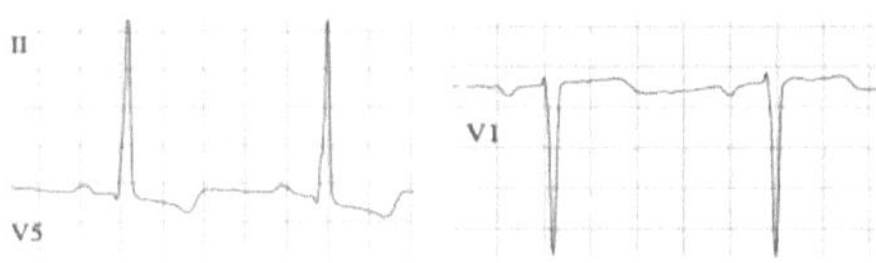

FIGURE 3.11

BIBLIOGRAPHY

1. O'Keefe, J. H., Pogwizd, S. M., Freed, M. S., & Hammill, S. C. (2015). *The ECG Criteria Book* (2nd ed.). Jones & Bartlett Learning.

Supraventricular and Junctional Rhythms

4

Ryan F. Heslin and Jahan Manjur

SUPRAVENTRICULAR RHYTHMS

Atrial Premature Beats

- Abnormal morphology P-wave with an early atrial depolarization relative to the normal PP interval
- QRS complex is usually similar in morphology

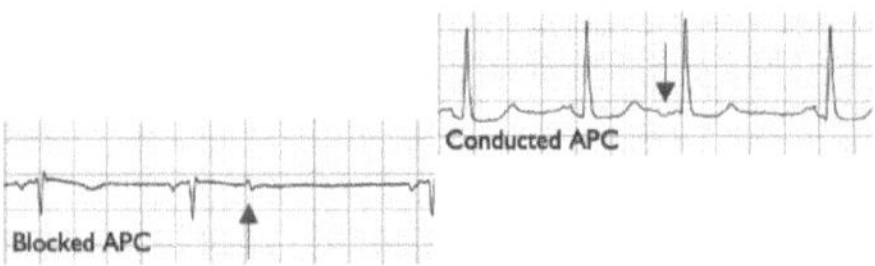

FIGURE 4.1

Exceptions

- Aberrantly conducted APCs (mostly RBBB-pattern)
- Blocked APCs (often buried in preceding T-wave)
  - Very premature P-wave not followed by a QRS

Atrial Tachycardia

- 3+ consecutive ectopic atrial beats (100–240 BPM)
- P-wave may precede, be buried in, or follow the QRS

DOI: 10.1201/9781003565383-4

- Has distinct isoelectric baseline between P-waves

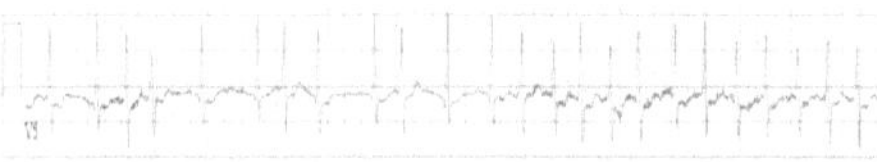

FIGURE 4.2

Multifocal AT

- 3+ P-wave morphologies [↓] with a rate >100 BPM
- If the rate is <100 BPM, termed "wandering pacemaker"
- Variable PP and PR intervals
- Conduction may be blocked or conducted with a narrow/wide QRS complex

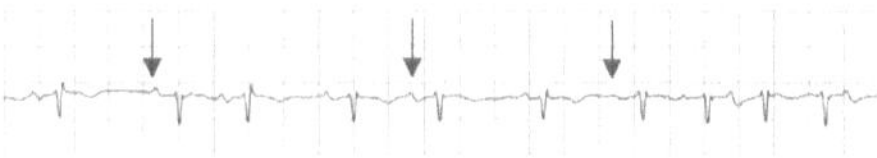

FIGURE 4.3

Atrial Fibrillation

- Discernible P-waves are absent, irregular atrial activity
- Fibrillatory ("f") waves of varying amplitude (coarse or fine), duration, morphology—random baseline oscillation
- Atrial activity is best seen in leads V_1, V_2, II, III, aVF
- Ventricular rhythm is typically irregularly irregular
- If the rate <100 BPM without AV blocking agents, there is likely underlying AV conduction system disease

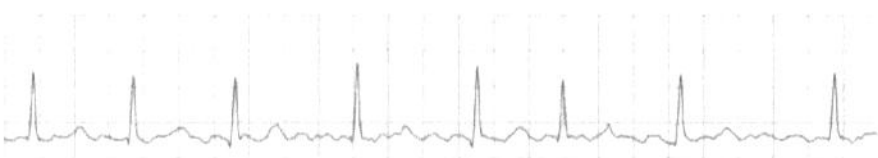

FIGURE 4.4

Atrial Flutter

- Rapid (240–340 BPM) and regular atrial undulations (flutter or "F" waves) in a sawtooth-like appearance
- QRS complex is normal or wide and commonly with a fixed even number (2:1, 4:1) ratio
- 4:1 block suggests AV conduction disease
- Flutter waves can deform QRS, ST, and/or T mimicking conduction delay and/or myocardial ischemia

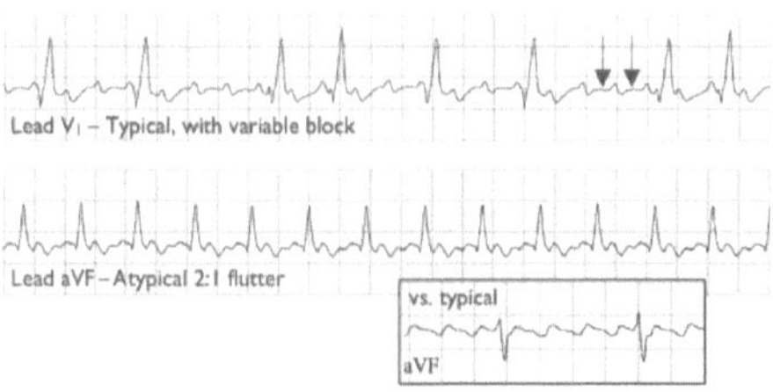

FIGURE 4.5

- **Typical Morphology**
  - *II/III/aVF*: <u>inverted</u> F waves <u>without</u> an isoelectric baseline
  - V_1: (+) deflections with a distinct isoelectric baseline [↓]
- **Atypical flutter can have upright F waves in II/III/aVF**

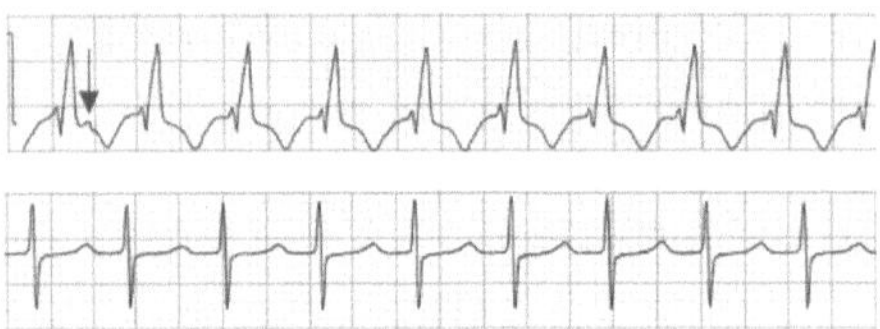

FIGURE 4.6

Paroxysmal SVT

- Unidentifiable P-waves with <u>regular</u> rhythm >100 BPM
- With or without aberrancy
  - Aberrancy results in WCT, mimicking VT
  - Differentiation is important; see VT section
- Abrupt onset/offset of dysrhythmia
- EP study to differentiate type of SVT

NB: In contrast to the other forms of atrial tachycardia, sinus node reentrant tachycardia manifests sinus P-waves and is indistinguishable from sinus tachycardia.

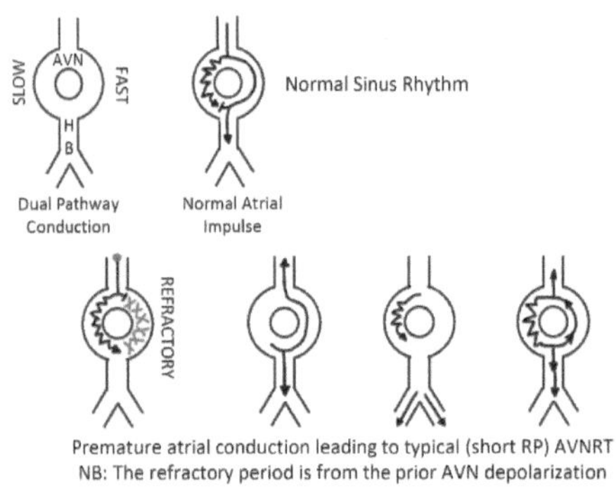

FIGURE 4.7

AV Nodal Reentrant Tachycardia

- Typical slow-fast AVNRT (85–90%)
  - Initiated by APC (when fast pathway isn't refractory)
  - Reentry occurs within the AV node:
    - Antegrade conduction = slow AV nodal pathway
    - Retrograde conduction = fast AV nodal pathway

  - Retrograde P-waves are often buried in the QRS (short RP), but may be present at the end of the QRS [↓] resulting in pseudo "r-prime" waves in V_1, V_2, or pseudo "s" waves in leads II, III, aVF
- Atypical AVNRT (10%)
  - Fast-slow or slow-slow (rare) AVNRT
  - Reentry circuit in AV node:
    - Antegrade = fast (or slow) AV node pathway
    - Retrograde conduction = slow AV node pathway
  - Retrograde P-waves are more commonly seen (long RP) in atypical AVNRT, after the QRS

AV Reentrant Tachycardia

- Reciprocating tachycardia over accessory pathway
- Most (90%) are orthodromic, retrograde via AP
- Occurs with WPW syndrome and other concealed bypass tracts
- Often initiated by APCs (blocking anterograde AP conduction and therefore allowing for subsequent retrograde conduction and perpetuation)
- Usually terminates suddenly

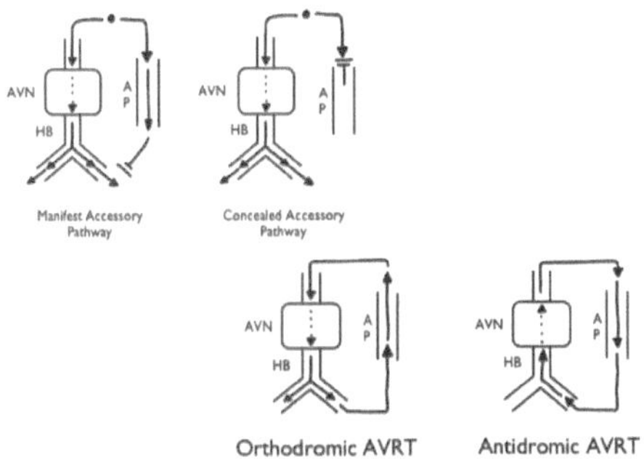

FIGURE 4.8

JUNCTIONAL RHYTHMS

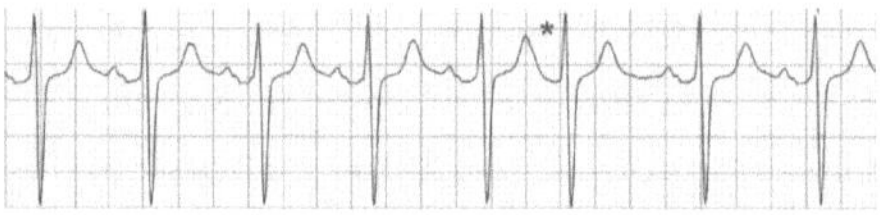

FIGURE 4.9

AV Junctional Premature Beats

- Premature QRS complex, narrow or wide
- P-wave may:
    - Precede the QRS by <110 ms (retrograde activation)
    - Be buried in the QRS complex (not visualized)
    - Follow the QRS complex
- Usually inverted P-waves in the inferior leads and upright in leads I and aVL due to atrial activation from near the AV node

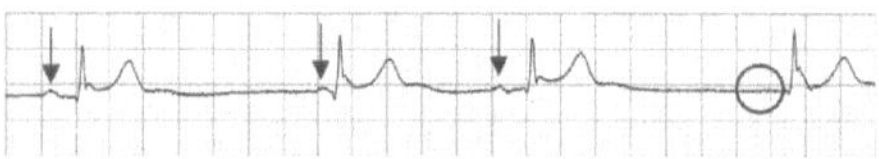

FIGURE 4.10

AV Junctional Escape Complex

- Typically narrow QRS that follow the previously conducted ventricular depolarization at a coupling interval rate of 40–60 BPM
- QRS morphology similar to sinus or supraventricular rhythm
- Usually a secondary phenomenon due to:
    - Decreased sinus impulse formation or conduction
    - High-degree AV block
    - Pause following termination of atrial dysrhythmia

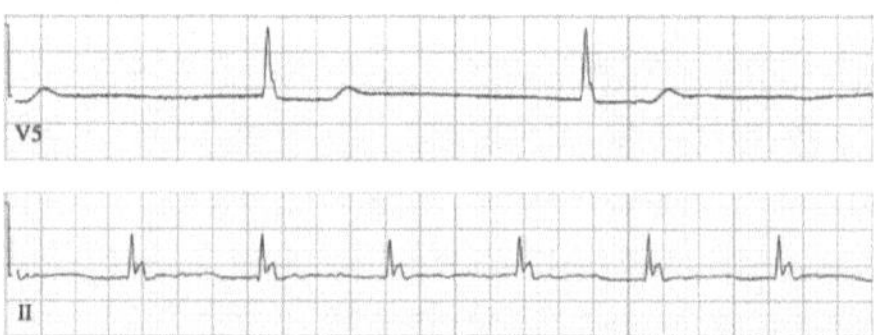

FIGURE 4.11

AV Junctional Rhythm/Tachycardia

- Regular rate of 40–60 BPM
- >60 BPM for junctional tachycardia
- Atrial and ventricular rates vary:
    - If retrograde (VA) block present, the atria remain in

sinus rhythm and AV dissociation will be present

- If retrograde atrial activation (inverted P waves in inferior leads) occurs, a constant QRS-P interval is usually present

BIBLIOGRAPHY

1. O'Keefe, J. H., Pogwizd, S. M., Freed, M. S., & Hammill, S. C. (2015). *The ECG Criteria Book* (2nd ed.). Jones & Bartlett Learning.

Ventricular Rhythms

5

Ryan F. Heslin and Jahan Manjur

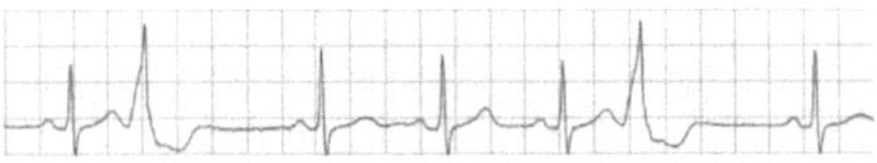

FIGURE 5.1

Ventricular Premature Complex (PVC)

- A wide, notched or slurred QRS
  - "Premature" relative to the normal RR interval
  - Not preceded by a P-wave (unless late-coupled sinus wave—PR interval <0.11 seconds)
  - QRS with initial deflection abnormal to baseline
- Secondary ST&T-wave changes:
  - Opposite to the major deflection of the QRS (i.e., ST depression and T-wave inversion in leads with a dominant R-wave and vice versa)
- Coupling interval may be constant or variable
- Morphology may be uniform or multiform
- A full compensatory pause (P-P containing the PVC is twice the normal PP interval)

DOI: 10.1201/9781003565383-5

Accelerated Idioventricular Rhythm

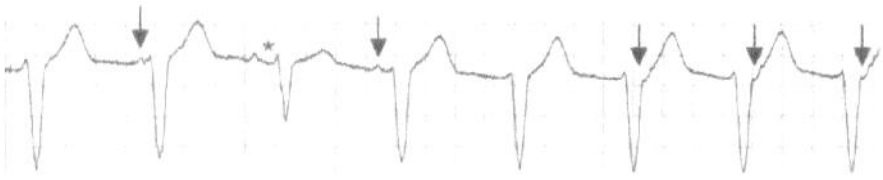

FIGURE 5.2

- Regular/slightly irregular ventricular (wide complex) rhythm at 60–110 BPM
- QRS morphology similar to PVCs
- AV dissociation [↓], ventricular capture complexes, and fusion beats [*] are common due to competing sinus and ectopic rhythms
- Seen after reperfusion, <u>not</u> prognostic

Ventricular Escape Complexes

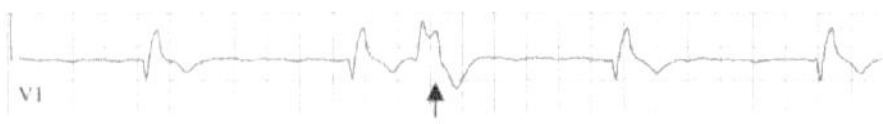

FIGURE 5.3

- Single beat or regular/slightly irregular ventricular rhythm at ~30–40 BPM
- QRS morphology can be similar to PVCs
- Escape may be a secondary to decreased sinus impulse formation/conduction, high-degree AV block, or after a conversion pause

Ventricular Tachycardia

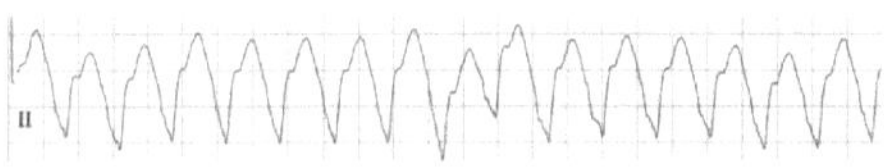

FIGURE 5.4

- 3+ PVCs with rate >100 BPM
  - "Sustained" if longer than 30 seconds
- RR is usually regular (but may be irregular)
- Monomorphic vs. Polymorphic vs. Biphasic
- AV dissociation common
- Retrograde atrial activation, fusion complex, and ventricular capture complexes may occur

DIFFERENTIATING VT AND SVT WITH ABERRANT CONDUCTION

Brugada Criteria (Accuracy 77%–85%)

- When NONE of the criteria are present, 15% still have VT

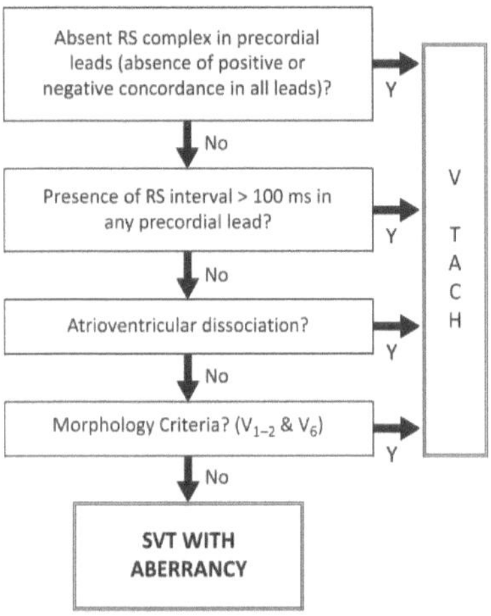

FIGURE 5.5

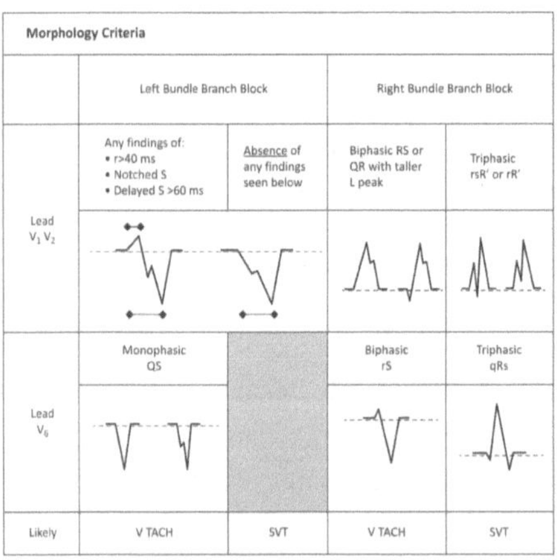

FIGURE 5.6

aVR Criteria

- Simplified, only looks at lead aVR

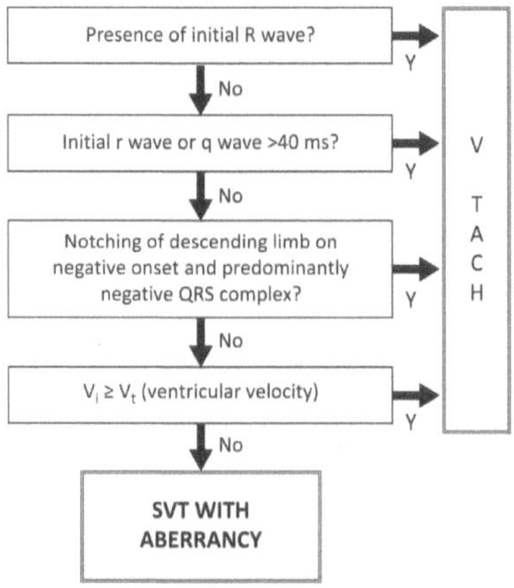

FIGURE 5.7

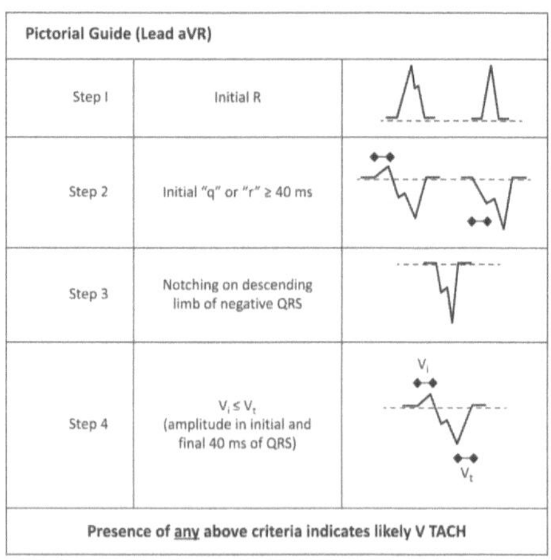

FIGURE 5.8

Torsades de Pointes

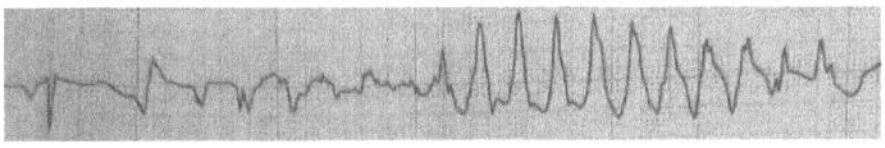

FIGURE 5.9

- **A subtype of polymorphic VT b/w 160**–250 BPM
- "Twisting of the points" as demonstrated by cycling of QRS axis within the same lead
- Usually seen in the context of QT prolongation, antecedent PVCs, and a compensatory pause
- Can degrade into ventricular fibrillation and sudden cardiac death

Ventricular Flutter

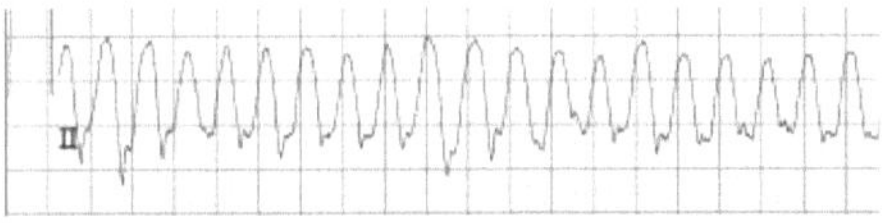

FIGURE 5.10

- Monomorphic ventricular tachycardia similar to ventricular fibrillation
- HR typically runs b/w 250–350 BPM
- Ventricular flutter lacks isoelectric intervals that lack clear QRS complexes, along with P and T waves
- Typically progresses to ventricular fibrillation, necessitating ACLS

Ventricular Fibrillation

- Unstable ventricular arrhythmia that is incompatible with life, most frequent rhythm in SCD
- Considered an "ischemic" rhythm, due to concurrence of underlying heart disease and myocardial hypoperfusion

- Over time, progresses from higher-amplitude "coarse" morphology to lower-amplitude "fine" ventricular fibrillation
- Rapid and irregular ventricular rhythm with:
  - Chaotic deflections of varying morphology
  - Absence of distinct P, QRS, and T waves
  - HR estimated at 300–500 BPM

BIBLIOGRAPHY

1. Brugada, P., Brugada, J., Mont, L., Smeets, J., & Andries, E. W. (1991, May 1). *A new approach to the differential diagnosis of a regular tachycardia with a wide QRS complex.* Circulation. https://pubmed.ncbi.nlm.nih.gov/2022022/
2. O'Keefe, J. H., Pogwizd, S. M., Freed, M. S., & Hammill, S. C. (2015). *The ECG Criteria Book* (2nd ed.). Jones & Bartlett Learning.
3. Vereckei, A. (2014, August). *Current algorithms for the diagnosis of wide QRS complex tachycardias.* Current cardiology reviews. https://www.ncbi.nlm.nih.gov/pmc/articles/PMC4040878/

Myocardial Ischemia, Injury, and Infarction

6

Ryan F. Heslin, Jahan Manjur, and On Chen

MYOCARDIAL INFARCTION

ECG Characteristics of Myocardial Damage

Ischemia (inadequate tissue oxygenation)

- ST-segment depression; usually TWI; Q-waves absent

Injury (prolonged ischemia)

- ST-segment elevation (compare to TP); Q-waves absent

Infarction (myocardial death)

- Abnormal Q-waves (may be present); STE or STD; T-waves inverted, normal, or upright & symmetrically peaked

DOI: 10.1201/9781003565383-6

ST Elevation Myocardial Infarction (STEMI)

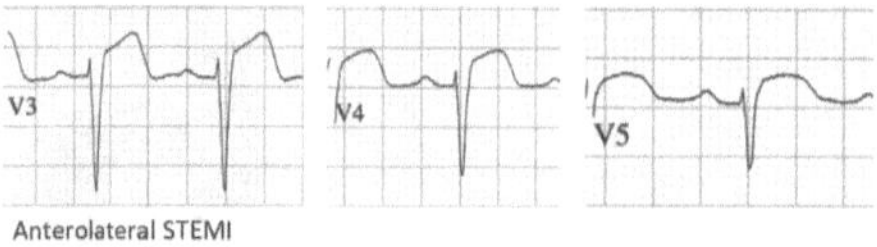

FIGURE 6.1

- New STE at the J ("junction") point in two contiguous leads
  - 2 mm in leads V_1, V_2, or V_3
  - 1 mm in other leads
- Usually upwardly convex ("tombstone") configuration
- Can persist 48 hours–4 weeks after MI
- Persistent STE >4 weeks suggests ventricular aneurysm
- TWI usually begins while ST segment is still elevated and may persist indefinitely

Pathological Q Wave

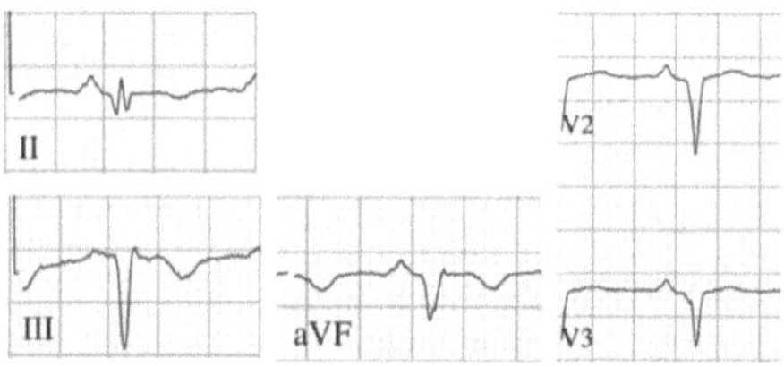

FIGURE 6.2

- Any Q wave ≥20 ms in leads V_2–V_3
- Q wave ≥30 ms and ≥0.1 mV in inferolateral leads
- R wave ≥40 ms in V_1–V_2 and R/S ≥1 with concordant (+) T-wave
- Must be present in 2+ contiguous leads
- Q-wave can't distinguish transmural vs. subendocardial MI

Age of Infarct

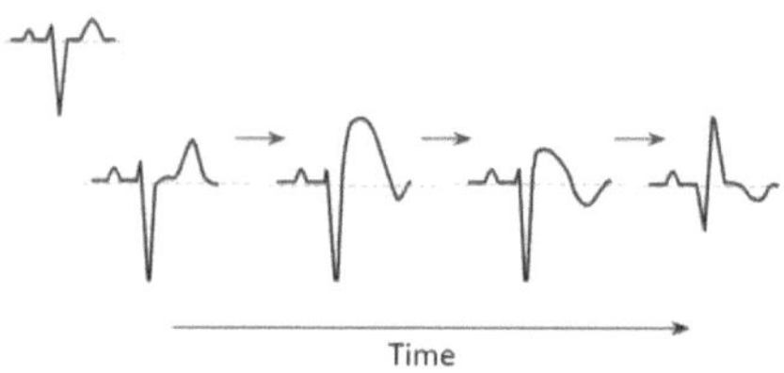

FIGURE 6.3

- The repolarization abnormalities associated with AMI typically evolve in a relatively predictable fashion
- Earliest findings include marked peaking of ("hyperacute") T-waves; often missed (occurring <15 minutes, transient)
- If transmural ischemia persists for more than minutes, peaked T-waves evolve into ST-segment elevation

- As infarction continues to evolve, the STE decreases, and the T-waves begin to invert (become progressively deeper)
- Abnormal Q-waves develop within the first few hours-days

Diagnosis of MI in Bundle Branch Blocks

- *RBBB*: *Does not interfere* with the diagnosis of MI
- *LBBB*: Difficult to diagnose any infarct if present

CORONARY ANATOMY

LOCATION	ST ELEVATION	RECIPROCAL CHANGES
Septal	V_1, V_2	–
Anterior	V_3, V_4	–
Anteroseptal	V_{1-4}	–
Lateral	I, aVL, V_5, V_6	II, III, aVF
Anterolateral	I, aVL, V_{3-6}	II, III, aVF
Inferior	II, III, aVF	I, aVL
Posterior	–	V_{1-4}

FIGURE 6.4

ECG localization of myocardial infarction			
I Lateral LCX	aVR – –	V_1 Septal LAD	V_4 Anterior LAD
II **Inferior** RCA (80%)/LCX (20%)	aVL Lateral LCX	V_2 Septal LAD	V_5 Lateral LCX
III **Inferior** RCA (80%)/LCX (20%)	aVF **Inferior** RCA (80%)/LCX (20%)	V_3 Anterior LAD	V_6 Lateral LCX

FIGURE 6.5

BIBLIOGRAPHY

1. O'Keefe, J. H., Pogwizd, S. M., Freed, M. S., & Hammill, S. C. (2015). *The ECG Criteria Book* (2nd ed.). Jones & Bartlett Learning.

Selected Clinical Disorders

7

Ryan F. Heslin, Jahan Manjur, and Mark Jacobs

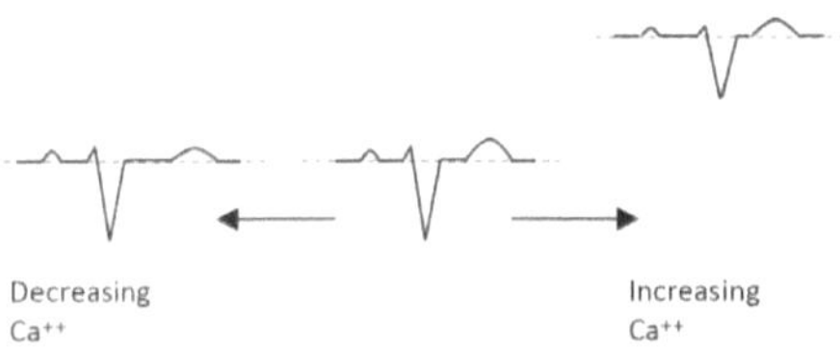

FIGURE 7.1

Hypercalcemia

- QTc shortening (due to shortening of the ST-segment)
- Potential PR prolongation

Hypocalcemia

- Prolonged QTc (earliest and most common finding) due to ST prolongation without changing duration of T-wave (only hypocalcemia or hypothermia)
- Occasional flattening, peaking, or inversion of T-waves

Acute Pericarditis

- Classic evolutionary ST and T-wave pattern in four stages:
  - *Stage I*: Upwardly concave non-reciprocal STE except aVR (STD)
  - *Stage II*: J point returns to baseline and T-wave amplitude decreases
  - *Stage III*: T-waves invert
  - *Stage IV*: ECG returns to normal

DOI: 10.1201/9781003565383-7

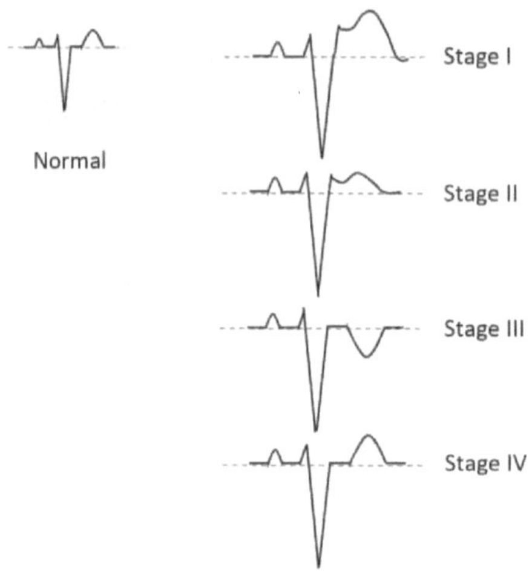

FIGURE 7.2

- TWI occurs after the ST returns to baseline (*unlike in myocardial infarction)
- Pericarditis may be focal (i.e., post-pericardiotomy) and result in regional (rather than diffuse) ST elevations
- Other features include: Sinus tachycardia, PR depression (elevation in aVR), and ECGs of pericardial effusion

Hypertrophic Cardiomyopathy

- Abnormal QRS (large amplitude, abnormal Q waves—pseudo-infarct pattern, and tall R waves with TWI in V_1—similar to RVH)
- Left axis deviation may be present
- ST and T wave changes (nonspecific, secondary to hypertrophy or conductional abnormalities; an apical variant of HCM manifests with deep TWI in V_4–V_6)
- LAE is common, RAE is occasionally present
- The most frequent cause of mortality is SCD (risk factors: Young age, history of syncope, and/or asymptomatic VT on ambulatory monitoring)

Digitalis Effect/Toxicity

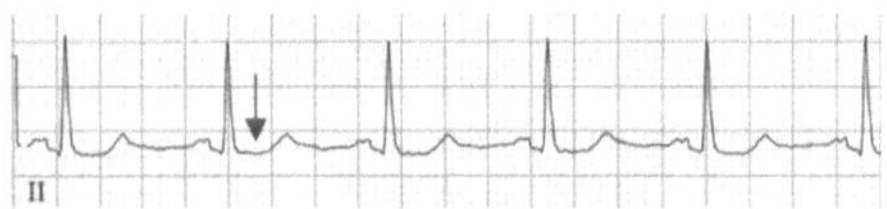

FIGURE 7.3

- Sagging (scooped out) ST-segment depression with upward concavity [↓]
- T-wave flat, inverted, or biphasic
- QT interval shortened

- U-wave amplitude increased
- PR interval lengthened
- With toxicity, almost any type of cardiac dysrhythmia or conduction disturbance is possible (except bundle branch block)
- Exacerbated by hypokalemia, hypomagnesemia, and hypercalcemia

NB: Electrical cardioversion of AF is contraindicated in digitalis toxicity since protracted asystole or ventricular fibrillation can occur

Anti-arrhythmic Drug Effect/Toxicity

- *Many effects*: Prominent U-waves (one of the earliest findings), QT prolongation, nonspecific ST and/or T-wave abnormalities, decrease in atrial flutter rate
- *Toxicity may lead to*: Severe QT prolongations, ventricular arrhythmias, wide QRS complex, various types of AV block, marked sinus bradycardia, sinus arrest, or sinoatrial exit block

Hyperkalemia

ECG changes depend on serum K+ level and slope of rise

- K+ = 5.5–6.5 mEq/L
  - Tall, peaked, narrow-based T-waves (generally >10 mm in precordial, >6 mm in limb leads) but is nonspecific
  - Reversible LAFB or LPFB

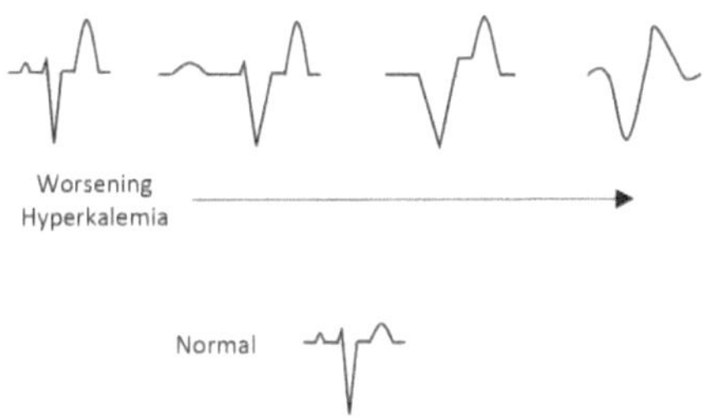

FIGURE 7.4

- K+ = 6.5–7.5 mEq/L
  - First-degree AV block
  - Flattening and widening of the P-wave, QRS widening
- K+ >7.5 mEq/L
  - Disappearance of P-waves
  - LBBB, RBBB, or sine-wave pattern
  - ST-segment elevation
  - Arrhythmias including VT, VF, idioventricular rhythm, asystole

Hypokalemia

- *Many effects*: Prominent U-waves, ST depression and flattened T-waves, increased amplitude and duration of P-wave, prolonged QT, arrhythmias including pAT with block, 1°/2° AV block, AV dissociation, PVCs, VT, and VF
- The ST-T and U-wave changes in ~80% with K+ <2.7 mEq/L, and only in 35% with 2.7–3.0 mEq/L

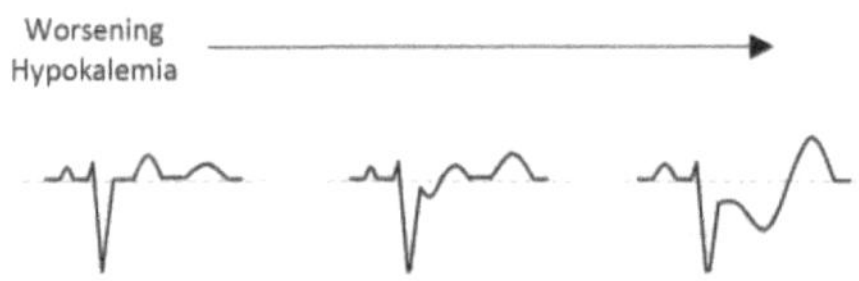

FIGURE 7.5

Central Nervous System Disorder

- "Classic changes" of cerebral and subarachnoid hemorrhage usually occur in the precordial leads:
  - Large upright or deeply inverted T-waves
  - Prolonged QT interval (often marked)
  - Prominent U-waves
- *Other changes*: T-wave notching, loss of T-wave amplitude, diffuse or focal STE, STD, Q-waves abnormalities

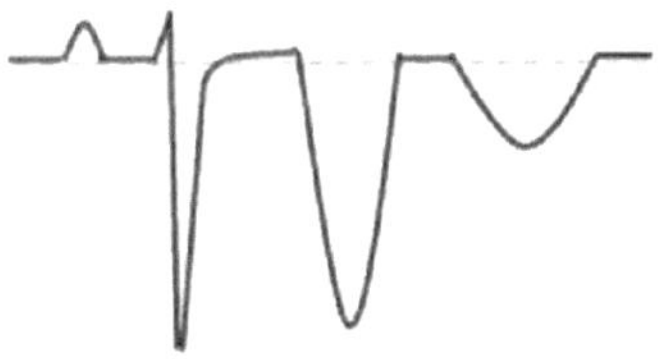

FIGURE 7.6

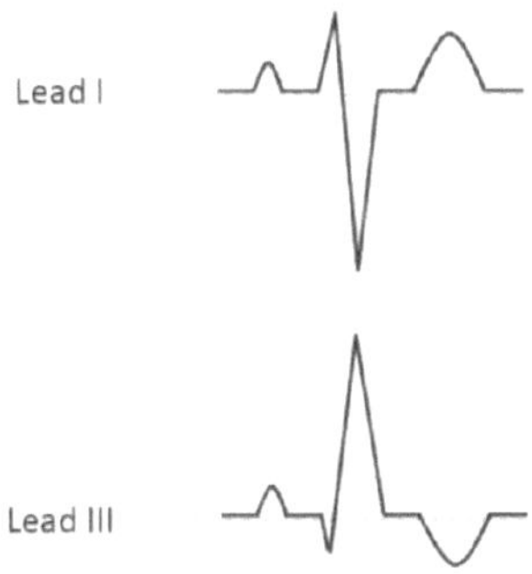

FIGURE 7.7

Chronic Lung Disease

- ECG features may include:
  - Right Atrial Enlargement
  - Poor precordial R-wave progression
  - Low voltage
  - Pseudo-anteroseptal infarct pattern (low anterior forces)
  - S1 S2 S3 pattern
  - Various conduction delays
- **RVH in chronic lung disease features—Rightward QRS shift, TWI in V_1, V_2, STD in inferior leads, transient RBBB, RSR or QR in V_1**

Acute Cor Pulmonale including Pulmonary Embolism

- ECG changes associated with elevated pulmonary artery pressures, right ventricular dilation and strain, and clockwise rotation
  - S_1Q_3 or $S_1Q_3T_3$ (~30%), lasting for 1–2 weeks
  - RBBB (~25%), complete or incomplete, lasting <1 week
  - TWI secondary to RV strain in R-sided precordial leads, lasting months
  - *Other features*: Right axis, nonspecific ST-T-wave changes, P. pulmonale
  - *Arrhythmias*: sinus tachycardia (most common), AF, flutter, AT, 1° AVB

NB: ECG findings of PE (QW/TWI) are similar to AWMI (can be distinguished by Q waves in lead II, which is uncommon in PE)

BIBLIOGRAPHY

1. O'Keefe, J. H., Pogwizd, S. M., Freed, M. S., & Hammill, S. C. (2015). *The ECG Criteria Book* (2nd ed.). Jones & Bartlett Learning.

Paced Rhythms

8

Ryan F. Heslin, Mark Jacobs, and Jahan Manjur

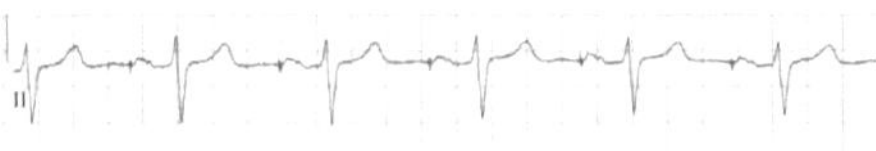

FIGURE 8.1

Atrial or Coronary Sinus Pacing

Pacemaker stimulus followed by an atrial depolarization

- If the rate of the intrinsic rhythm is less than the PM, atrial pacing occurs with a constant A-A
- Appropriately sensed intrinsic atrial activity resets programmed pacemaker timer

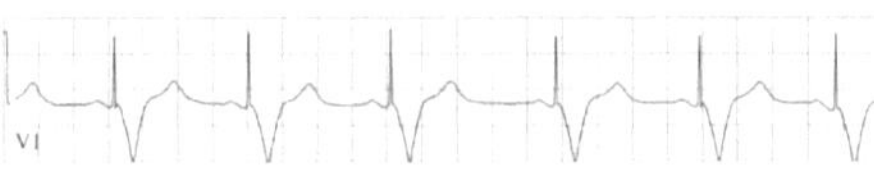

FIGURE 8.2

Ventricular Demand Pacemaker (VVI)

Pacemaker stimulus followed by a QRS of different morphology than native/baseline

- VVI pacemaker senses/paces only in the ventricle and is oblivious to native atrial activity
  - If constant ventricular pacing is noted throughout the tracing, it is impossible to distinguish ventricular demand from *asynchronous ventricular pacing*

DOI: 10.1201/9781003565383-8

- The diagnosis of ventricular demand pacing requires appropriate inhibition of PM output in response to at least one native QRS
- Appropriately sensed ventricular activity resets programmed pacemaker timer

Dual-Chamber Pacemaker

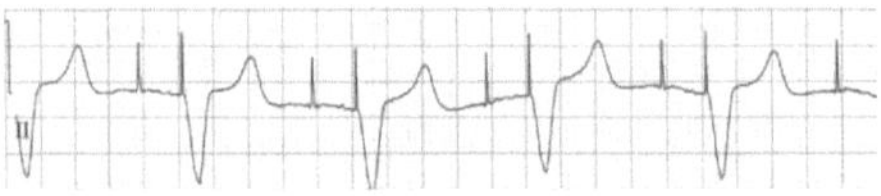

FIGURE 8.3

- Atrial and ventricular pacing and sensing
    - *Atrial sensing*: Needs to demonstrate inhibition of atrial output and/or triggering of ventricular stimulus in response to intrinsic atrial activity
- If pacemaker rate exceeds rate of intrinsic rhythm, there will be atrial (A) and ventricular (V) paced beats with defined A-V and V-A intervals
- Following V-sensed activity (QRS or paced beat), the programmed pacemaker timer resets
    - If intrinsic atrial activity (P) is sensed prior to end of V-A interval, atrial output of the PM will be inhibited
- Following A-sensed activity (intrinsic or paced beat), programmed pacemaker timer resets
    - If intrinsic ventricular activity (QRS) is sensed prior to end of A-V interval, ventricular output of the pacemaker should be inhibited

BIBLIOGRAPHY

1. O'Keefe, J. H., Pogwizd, S. M., Freed, M. S., & Hammill, S. C. (2015). *The ECG Criteria Book* (2nd ed.). Jones & Bartlett Learning.

9

Selected ECG Review*

Ryan F. Heslin, Abhijeet Singh, On Chen, and Andreas Kalogeropoulos

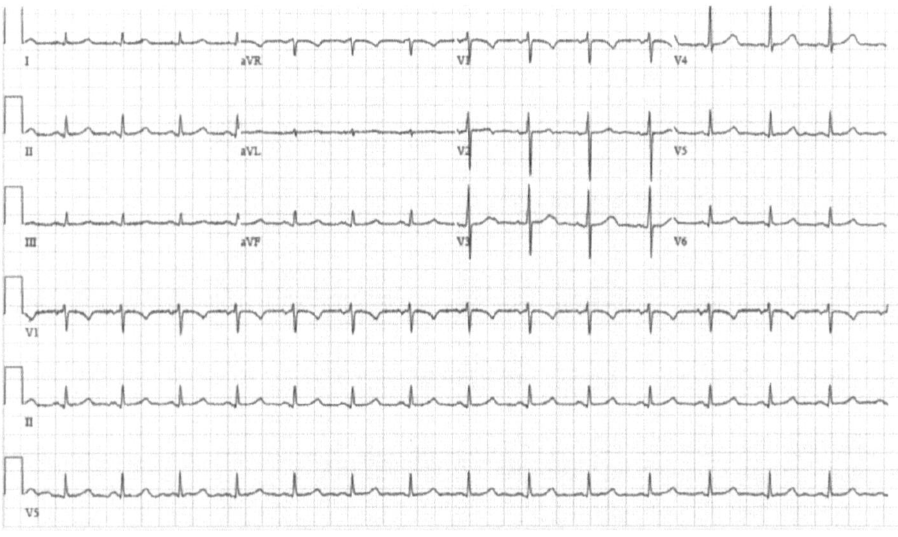

FIGURE 9.1

Rhythm: Sinus rhythm
Rate: 82 BPM
Axis: Normal (Physiologic)
Intervals: Normal

* A special acknowledgement goes to Ryan Heslin for his dedication and meticulous attention to detail in helping write and review over 100 ECG interpretations in this chapter.

P-wave: Normal
QRS Complex: Normal
T-wave: Normal
Infarct: None

This ECG demonstrates normal sinus rhythm (NSR), as the P-waves in Leads I, II, and aVF are positive, and the P-wave in Lead V1 is biphasic. The PR interval, QRS duration, ST segment, and TP interval are all normal in duration, and the waves and complexes contained within them are of normal morphology.

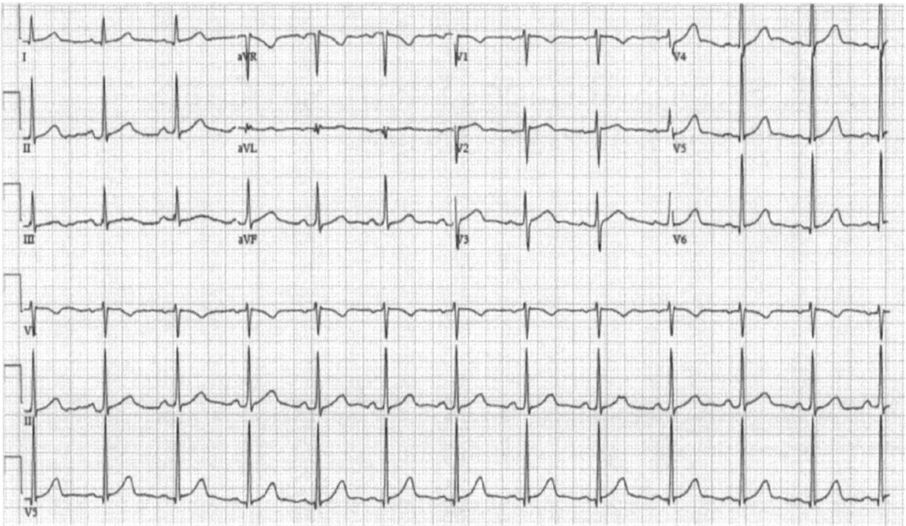

FIGURE 9.2

Rhythm: Sinus rhythm
Rate: 72 BPM
Axis: Normal (Physiologic)
Intervals: Normal
P-wave: Normal
QRS Complex: Normal
T-wave: Normal
Infarct: None

This ECG demonstrates normal sinus rhythm (NSR), as the P-waves in Leads I, II, and aVF are positive, and the P-wave in Lead V1 is biphasic. The PR interval, QRS duration, ST segment, and TP interval are all normal in duration, and the waves and complexes contained within them are of normal morphology.

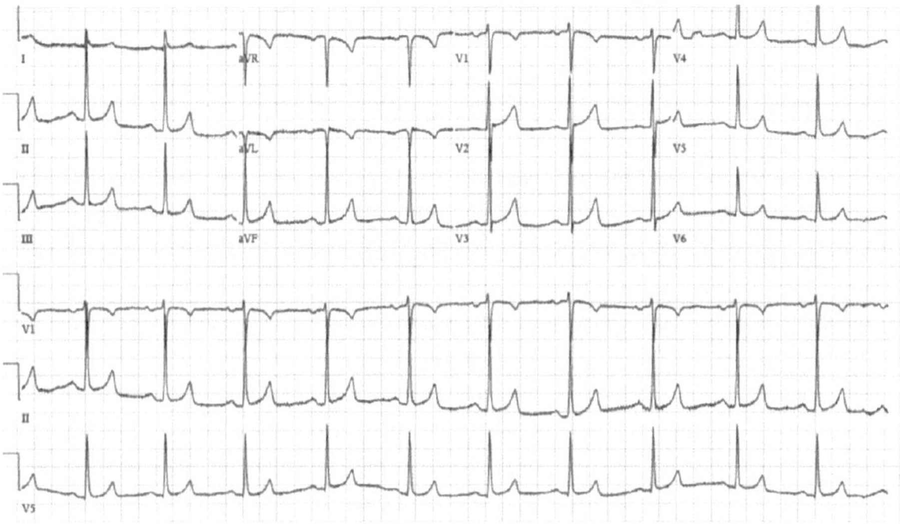

FIGURE 9.3

Rhythm: Sinus rhythm
Rate: 64 BPM
Axis: Normal (Physiologic)
Intervals: Normal
P-wave: Normal
QRS Complex: Normal
T-wave: Normal
Infarct: None

This ECG demonstrates normal sinus rhythm (NSR), as the P-waves in Leads I, II, and aVF are positive, and the P-wave in Lead V1 is biphasic. There is an early transition of forces along the precordial leads, with the R-wave in Lead V2 being greater in amplitude than its corresponding S-wave.

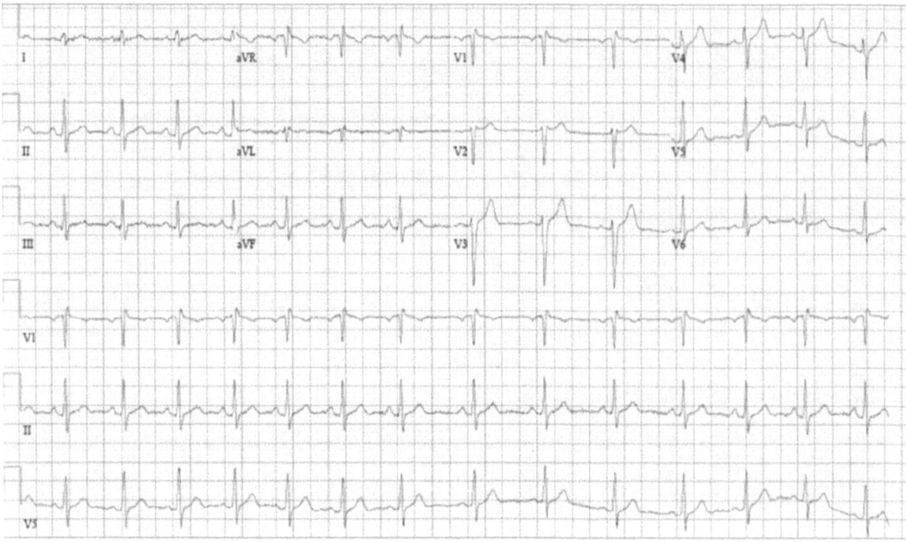

FIGURE 9.4

Rhythm: Sinus rhythm with sinus arrhythmia
Rate: 74 BPM
Axis: Normal (Physiologic)
Intervals: Normal
P-wave: Normal
QRS Complex: RV Conduction delay
T-wave: Normal
Infarct: None

This ECG demonstrates normal sinus rhythm (NSR), as the P-waves in Leads I, II, and aVF are positive. Sinus arrhythmia is present as well, which is defined as the presence of sinus rhythm with a >120 ms variation in the RR interval. The relative inhibition of vagal tone during inspiration enables an increase in heart rate (HR), with the physiology being reversed during exhalation. There is a right ventricular (RV) conduction delay present, as the QRS complex adopts a right bundle branch block (RBBB) morphology but is <100 ms in duration.

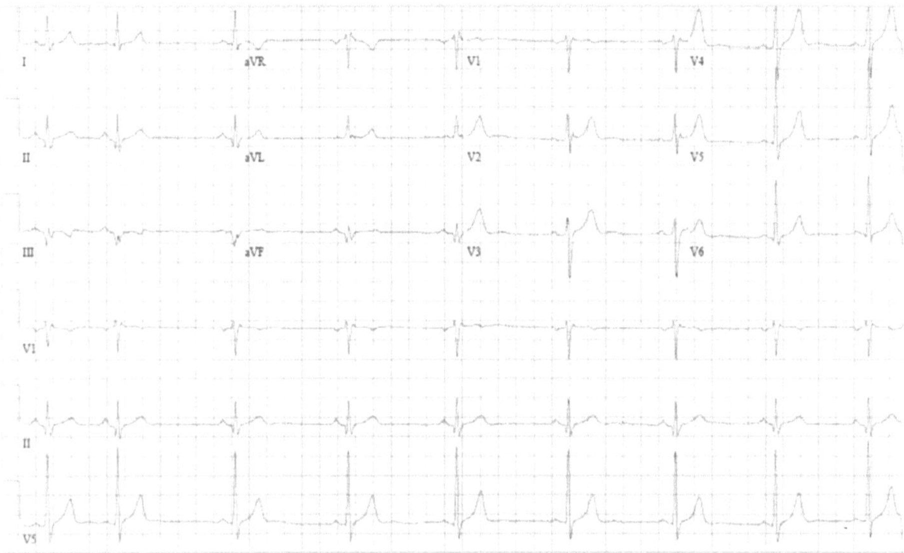

FIGURE 9.5

Rhythm: Sinus bradycardia
Rate: 54 BPM
Axis: Normal (Physiologic)
Intervals: Normal
P-wave: Normal
QRS Complex: Normal
T-wave: Normal
Infarct: Pathological Q-waves in Leads II, III, and aVF

This ECG demonstrates sinus rhythm as the P-waves in Leads I, II, and aVF are positive, and the P-wave in Lead V1 is biphasic. The rate <60 BPM is consistent with bradycardia. A premature atrial contraction (PAC) is present, as the 2nd P-wave has a slightly different morphology when compared to the other P-waves on the tracing. The pathological Q-waves in the Leads II, III, and aVF are likely indicative of an old myocardial infarction (MI). The QRS complex of Lead V2 is positive, even though the QRS complexes of Leads V1 and V3 are both negative, which is likely indicative of mispositioning of Lead V2.

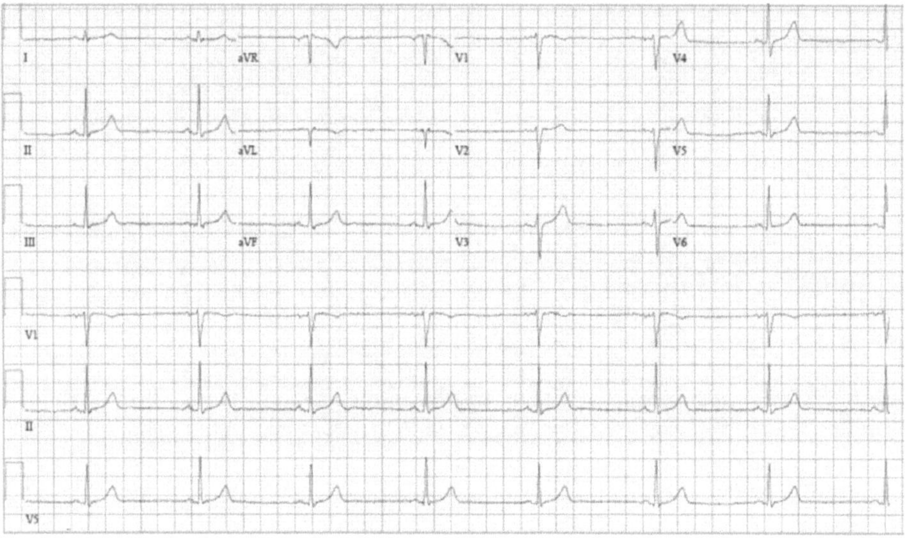

FIGURE 9.6

Rhythm: Sinus bradycardia
Rate: 48 BPM
Axis: Normal (Physiologic)
Intervals: Normal
P-wave: Normal
QRS Complex: Normal
T-wave: Normal
Infarct: None

This ECG demonstrates sinus rhythm as the P-waves in Leads I, II, and aVF are positive, and the P-wave in Lead V1 is biphasic. The rate <60 BPM is consistent with bradycardia. The PR interval, QRS duration, ST segment, and TP interval are all normal in duration, and the waves and complexes contained within them are of normal morphology.

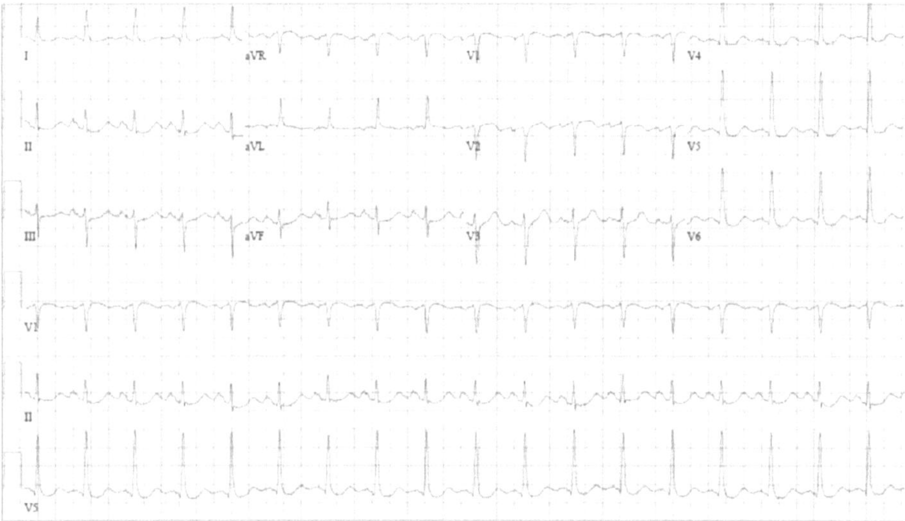

FIGURE 9.7

Rhythm: Sinus tachycardia
Rate: 108 BPM
Axis: Normal (Physiologic)
Intervals: Normal
P-wave: Normal
QRS Complex: Normal
T-wave: Nonspecific T-wave abnormality along Leads I, II, aVL, and V4–V6
Infarct: None

This ECG demonstrates sinus rhythm as the P-waves in Leads I, II, and aVF are positive, and the P-wave in Lead V1 is biphasic. The rate >100 BPM is consistent with tachycardia. There is a nonspecific T-wave abnormality along Leads I, II, aVL, and V4–V6, most prominently in the lateral leads.

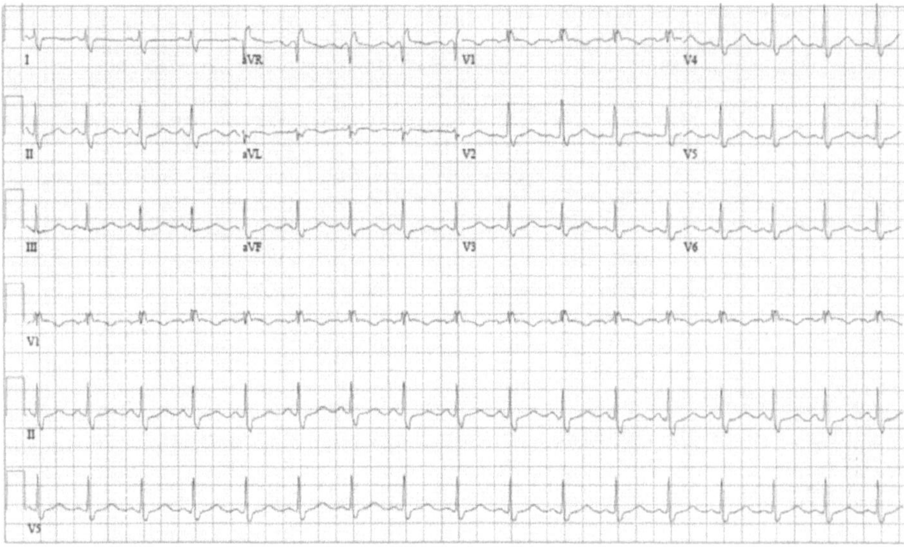

FIGURE 9.8

Rhythm: Sinus tachycardia
Rate: 101 BPM
Axis: Right axis deviation (RAD)
Intervals: Normal
P-wave: Normal
QRS Complex: Incomplete right bundle branch block (iRBBB)
T-wave: T-wave flattening in Leads I and aVL
Infarct: None

This ECG demonstrates sinus rhythm as the P-waves in Leads I, II, and aVF are positive, and the P-wave in Lead V1 is biphasic. The rate >100 BPM is consistent with tachycardia. An rSR' morphology is present in Lead V1 in conjunction with a QRS complex of <120 ms in duration. This is indicative of an incomplete right bundle branch block (incomplete RBBB). Furthermore, a right axis deviation (RAD) is present, as the S-wave in Lead I is greater in amplitude than the corresponding R-wave, while the QRS complex in Leads II and aVF are positive in amplitude. There is a nonspecific T-wave abnormality, most consistent with flattening in Leads I and aVL.

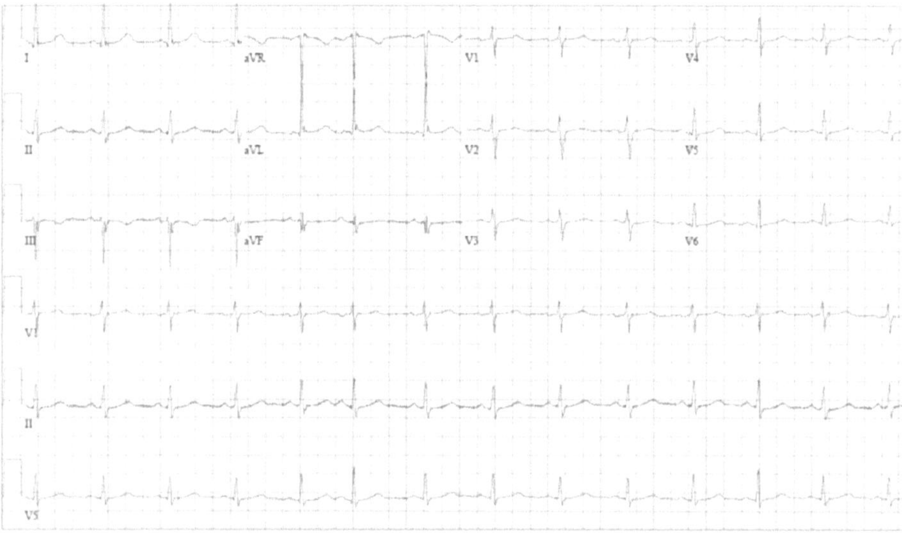

FIGURE 9.9

Rhythm: Sinus rhythm
Rate: 82 BPM
Axis: Normal (Physiologic)
Intervals: Normal
P-wave: Normal
QRS Complex: Normal
T-wave: Nonspecific T-wave flattening along Leads III, V2, and V3
Infarct: None

This ECG demonstrates normal sinus rhythm (NSR), as the P-waves in Leads I, II, and aVF are positive, and the P-wave in Lead V1 is biphasic. The PR interval, QRS duration, ST segment, and TP interval are all normal in duration, and the waves and complexes contained within them are of normal morphology. A premature atrial complex (PAC) is present and is best seen as the 6th beat on the rhythm strip. The PAC is indicative of an atrial depolarization (and subsequent ventricular depolarization that engages the His Bundle) that comes from a different focus, resulting in a decreased RR interval. Non-interpolated PACs will be followed by a compensatory pause prior to the next normal sinus beat (7th beat) parking the return to normal conduction. There is nonspecific T-wave flattening along Leads III, V2, and V3.

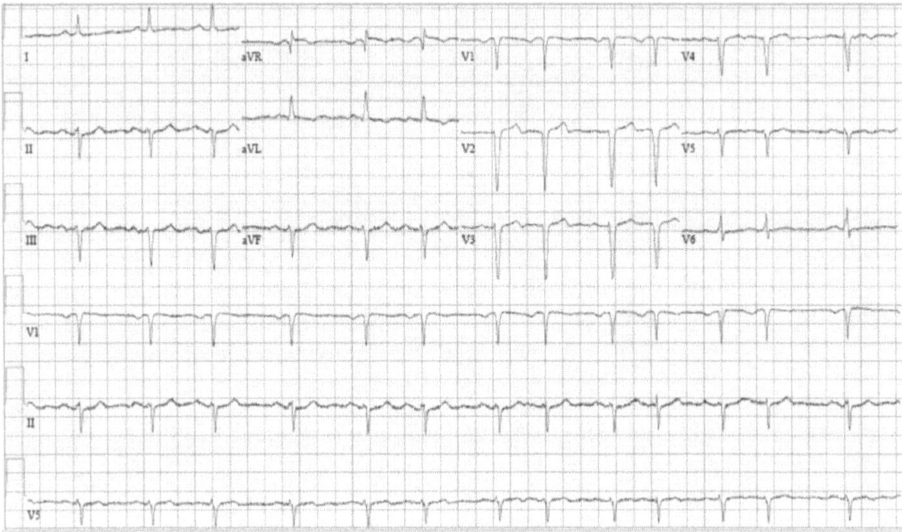

FIGURE 9.10

Rhythm: Sinus rhythm
Rate: 79 BPM
Axis: Left axis deviation (LAD)
Intervals: Normal
P-wave: Normal
QRS Complex: Pathological Q-waves in Leads V1–V3
T-wave: Nonspecific T-wave flattening in Leads I, aVL, V1, V5, and V6
Infarct: Prior anteroseptal myocardial infarction

This ECG demonstrates normal sinus rhythm (NSR), as the P-waves in Leads I, II, and aVF are positive. There are frequent PACs, best appreciated on the rhythm strip as the 6th, 8th, 10th, and 12th beats. This specific pattern is consistent with a salvo of atrial bigeminy, in which a sinus beat is followed by a PAC, then by a compensatory pause before the next sinus beat comes through. This tracing shows wide, pathological Q-waves in Leads V1–V3, concerning for a previous anterior wall myocardial infarction (MI) of unknown (although not acute) age. There is a left axis deviation (LAD) present in this ECG as well, as indicated by the R-wave amplitude > S-wave amplitude in Lead I, in contrast to the R-wave amplitude < S-wave amplitude in Lead II. There is an associated poor R-wave progression (PRWP) along the precordial leads, as the QRS complex does not become positive until Lead V6, with the isoelectric point between Leads V5 and V6. Also noted is nonspecific T-wave flattening in Leads I, aVL, V1, V5, and V6.

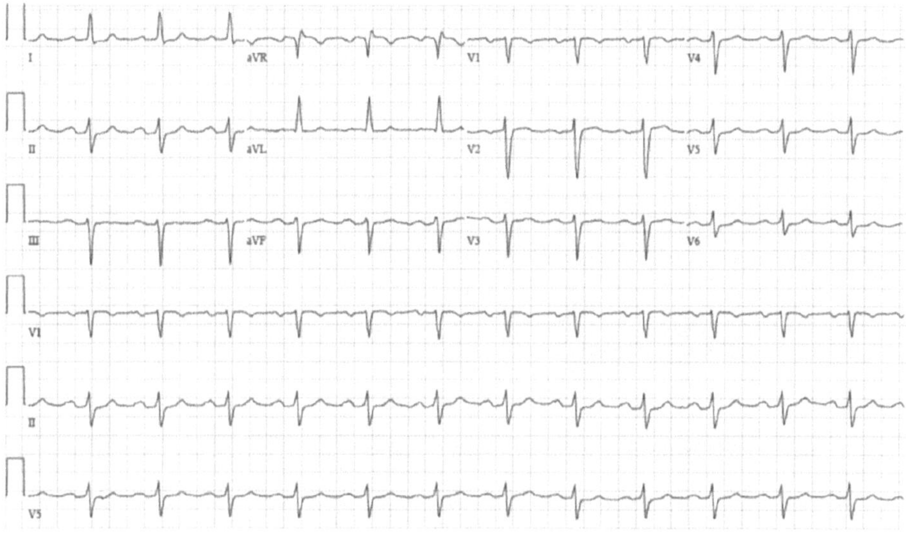

FIGURE 9.11

Rhythm: Sinus rhythm
Rate: 77 BPM
Axis: Left axis deviation (LAD)
Intervals: PR interval >200 ms (1st Degree AV delay)
P-wave: Left atrial abnormality (LAA)
QRS Complex: Poor R-wave progression (PRWP)
T-wave: Nonspecific T-wave flattening in Lead III
Infarct: None

This ECG demonstrates normal sinus rhythm (NSR), as the P-waves in Leads I, II, and aVF are positive, and the P-wave in Lead V1 is biphasic. The P-wave duration is borderline at ~120 ms, and the P-wave in Lead II demonstrates "notching (P-mitrale)," suggesting a left atrial abnormality (LAA) is present. The PR interval is >200 ms, which is indicative of a 1st degree atrioventricular (AV) delay. There are nonspecific T-waves changes, namely T-wave flattening, evident in Leads III and aVF. Note that a 1st degree AV delay is not referred to as an AV block in this text because a QRS is not "dropped," as would be the case with higher-degree blocks. There is a left axis deviation (LAD) present in this ECG as well, as indicated by the R-wave amplitude > S-wave amplitude in Lead I, in contrast to the R-wave amplitude < S-wave amplitude in Lead II. There is an associated poor R-wave progression (PRWP) along the precordial leads, as the QRS complex does not become positive until Lead V6, with the isoelectric point between Leads V5 and V6.

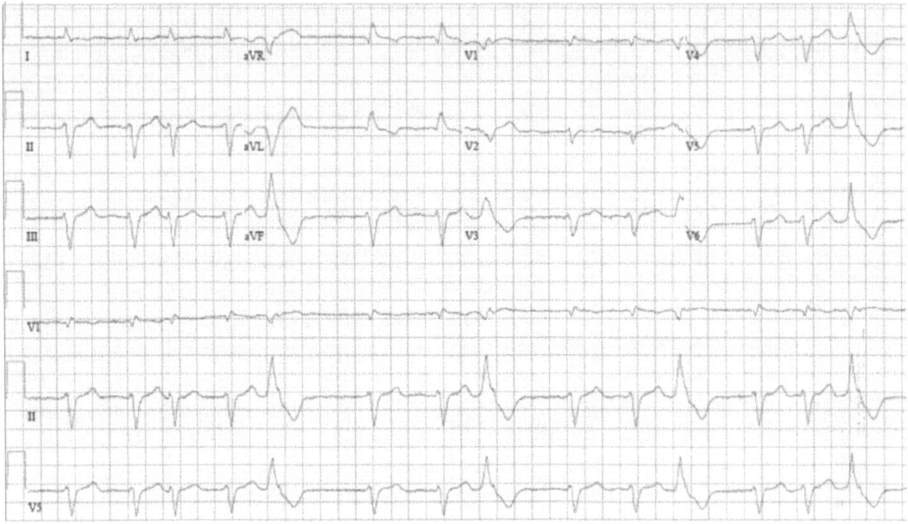

FIGURE 9.12

Rhythm: Atrial fibrillation with a controlled ventricular response (CVR)
Rate: 84 BPM
Axis: Left axis deviation (LAD)
Intervals: QRS Complex duration ~120 ms
P-wave: Not applicable
QRS Complex: Right bundle branch block (RBBB)
T-wave: T-wave inversions (TWIs) along Leads I and aVL
Infarct: None

This ECG demonstrates f-waves rather than P-waves, which is indicative of atrial fibrillation (Afib). The atrial rate being >300 beats per minute (BPM) and the different morphologies of the f-waves within any given lead also denote Afib. With a ventricular rate between 60 BPM and 100 BPM, as is the case with this tracing, the proper terminology would be Afib with a controlled ventricular response (CVR). The patient has frequent premature ventricular complexes (PVCs), which are best appreciated on the rhythm strip as the 5th, 8th, 11th, and 14th beats. This particular pattern is consistent with ventricular trigeminy, in which two consecutive sinus beats are followed by a PVC, then by a compensatory pause before the next sinus beat comes through. A PVC is indicative of a ventricular depolarization, which travels retrograde up the His Bundle, causing a wide-QRS beat that interrupts the cardiac cycle. There is a left axis deviation (LAD) present in this ECG as well, as indicated by the R-wave amplitude > S-wave amplitude in Lead I, in contrast to the R-wave amplitude < S-wave amplitude in Lead II. An rSR' is present in Lead V1, and the QRS complex is >120 ms in duration, which is consistent with a right bundle branch block (RBBB). There are T-wave inversions (TWIs) along Leads I and aVL. There is an associated poor R-wave progression (PRWP) along the precordial leads, as the QRS complex does not become positive by Lead V6.

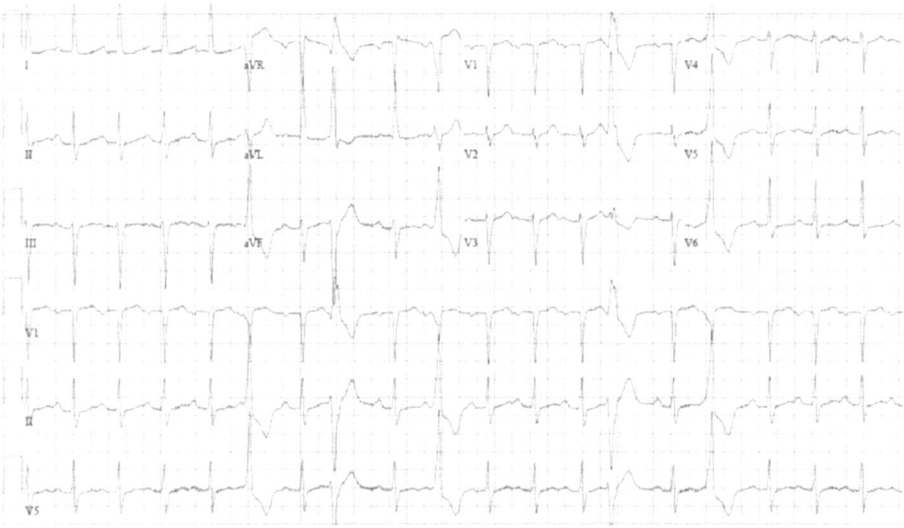

FIGURE 9.13

Rhythm: Sinus tachycardia
Rate: 119 BPM
Axis: Normal (Physiologic)
Intervals: PR-interval >200 ms (1st Degree AV delay)
P-wave: Normal
QRS Complex: Normal
T-wave: Normal
Infarct: None

This ECG demonstrates sinus rhythm as the P-waves in Leads I, II, and aVF are positive, and the P-wave in Lead V1 is biphasic. The rate >100 BPM is consistent with tachycardia. There are multiple PVCs present on this tracing. These PVCs are best appreciated as the 6th, 8th, 14th, and 16th beats. The PVCs are multifocal—with beats 6 and 16 adopting a left bundle morphology and beats 8 and 14 adopting a right bundle morphology. There is also a prolonged PR-interval >200 ms, which is consistent with a 1st degree AV delay.

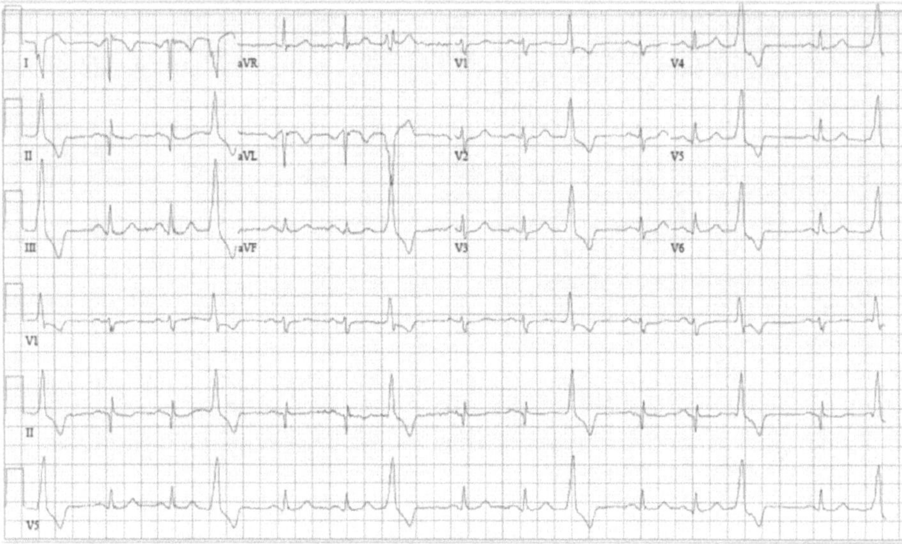

FIGURE 9.14

Rhythm: Sinus rhythm with ventricular trigeminy
Rate: 90 BPM
Axis: Right axis deviation (RAD)
Intervals: PR interval ~200 ms (1st Degree AV delay)
P-wave: Normal
QRS Complex: Normal
T-wave: T-wave inversions (TWIs) in Lead II
Infarct: None

This ECG demonstrates sinus rhythm as the P-waves in Leads II, III, and aVF are positive. This particular pattern is consistent with ventricular trigeminy, in which two consecutive sinus beats are followed by a PVC, then by a compensatory pause before the next sinus beat comes through. A PVC is indicative of a ventricular depolarization, which travels retrograde up the His Bundle, causing a wide-QRS beat that interrupts the cardiac cycle. The QRS axis on this tracing is likely borderline between a RAD (due to the negative QRS amplitude in Lead I) and a Northwestern axis (due to the S-wave in Lead II being > in amplitude than the corresponding R-wave). There is also a borderline 1st degree AV delay, due to the PR interval approaching 200 ms in duration. There is a T-wave inversion (TWI) in Lead II. Additionally, the QRS complex polarity is positive in Lead aVR and negative in Lead aVL, which would imply a lead switch between the left and right arm leads.

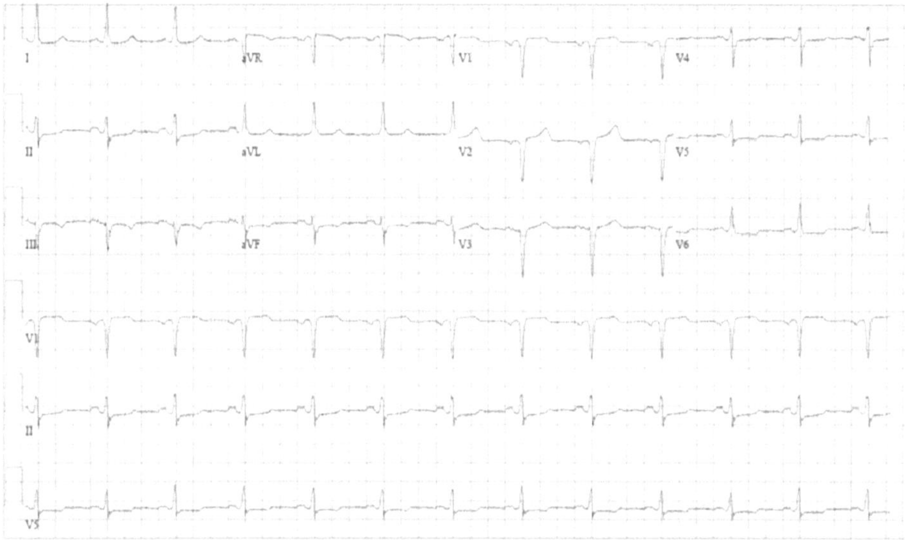

FIGURE 9.15

Rhythm: Sinus rhythm
Rate: 75 BPM
Axis: Normal (Physiologic)
Intervals: ST-segment depressions in Leads III, aVF, V5, and V6
P-wave: Left atrial abnormality (LAA)
QRS Complex: Pathological Q-waves in Leads V1–V3; Poor R-wave progression (PRWP)
T-wave: T-wave inversions (TWIs) and ST-segment depressions in Leads III, aVF, V5, and V6
Infarct: Prior anteroseptal wall myocardial infarction

This ECG demonstrates normal sinus rhythm (NSR) as the P-waves in Leads I, II, and aVF are positive, and the P-wave in Lead V1 is biphasic. The deep terminal aspect of the P-wave in Lead V1, P-wave duration >120 ms in Lead II, and P-wave notching (P-mitrale) points to a left atrial abnormality (LAA). This tracing also shows wide, pathological Q-waves in Leads V1–V3, concerning for a previous anterior wall myocardial infarction (MI) of unknown (although not acute) age. There is an associated poor R-wave progression (PRWP) along the precordial leads, as the QRS complex does not become positive until Lead V5, with the isoelectric point between Leads V4 and V5. There are T-wave inversions (TWIs) and ST-segment depressions in Leads III, aVF, V5, and V6.

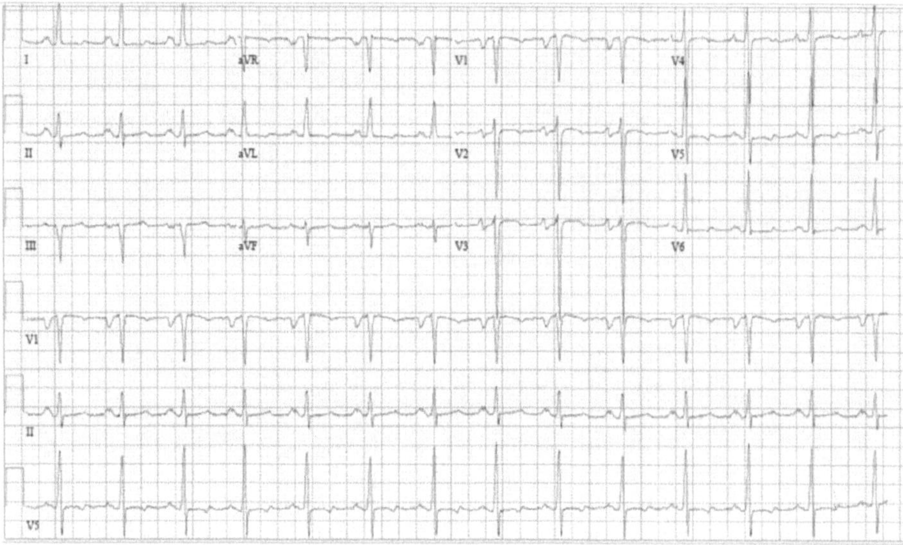

FIGURE 9.16

Rhythm: Sinus rhythm
Rate: 83 BPM
Axis: Normal (Physiologic)
Intervals: Normal
P-wave: Left atrial abnormality (LAA)
QRS Complex: Poor R-wave progression (PRWP); Left ventricular hypertrophy (LVH)
T-wave: Nonspecific T-wave flattening along Leads V1–V4
Infarct: None

This ECG demonstrates normal sinus rhythm (NSR) as the P-waves in Leads I, II, and aVF are positive, and the P-wave in Lead V1 is biphasic. Due to the terminal component of the biphasic P-wave in Lead V1 being ~2.5 small boxes deep and two small boxes wide (~2.5 mm deep and ~80 ms wide), a left atrial abnormality (LAA) is present. This is further supported by P-mitrale, a notching of the P-wave that is present in Lead II. Poor R-wave progression (PRWP) is present along the precordial leads, as the QRS complex does not become positive (aside from Lead V1) until Lead V5, with the isoelectric point between Leads V4 and V5. There is nonspecific T-wave flattening along Leads V1–V4. Based upon the modified Cornell criteria, the R-wave >11 mm in amplitude in Lead aVL is indicative of left ventricular hypertrophy (LVH).

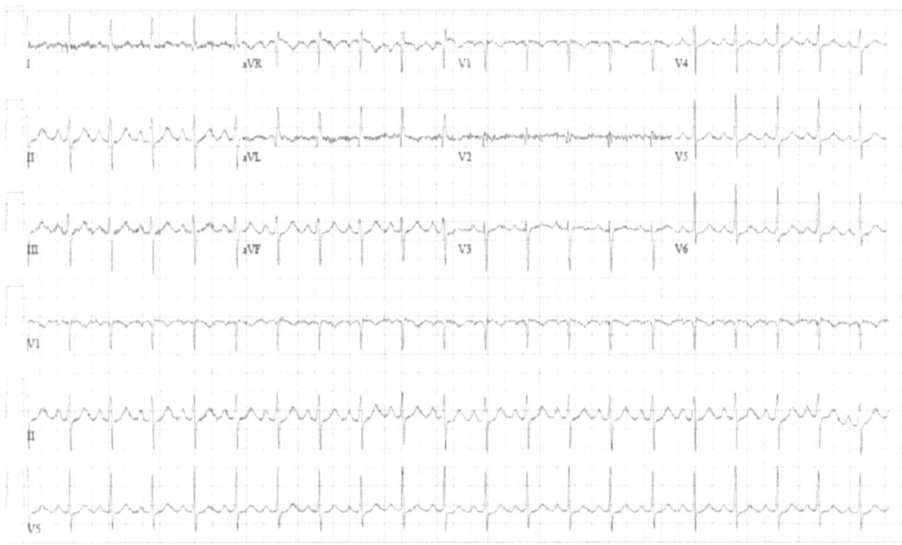

FIGURE 9.17

Rhythm: Sinus tachycardia
Rate: 126 BPM
Axis: Left axis deviation (LAD)
Intervals: Normal
P-wave: Right atrial abnormality (RAA)
QRS Complex: Normal
T-wave: Normal
Infarct: None

This ECG demonstrates sinus rhythm as the P-waves in Leads II, III, and aVF are positive. The rate >100 BPM is consistent with tachycardia. The P-wave in Lead II is consistent with "P-pulmonale," insofar as it is >2.5 mm in amplitude; all three of the inferior leads (Leads II, III, and aVF) display a similar morphology. This pattern is consistent with a right atrial abnormality (RAA). There is a left axis deviation (LAD) present in this ECG as well, as indicated by the R-wave amplitude > S-wave amplitude in Lead I, in contrast to the R-wave amplitude < S-wave amplitude in Lead II.

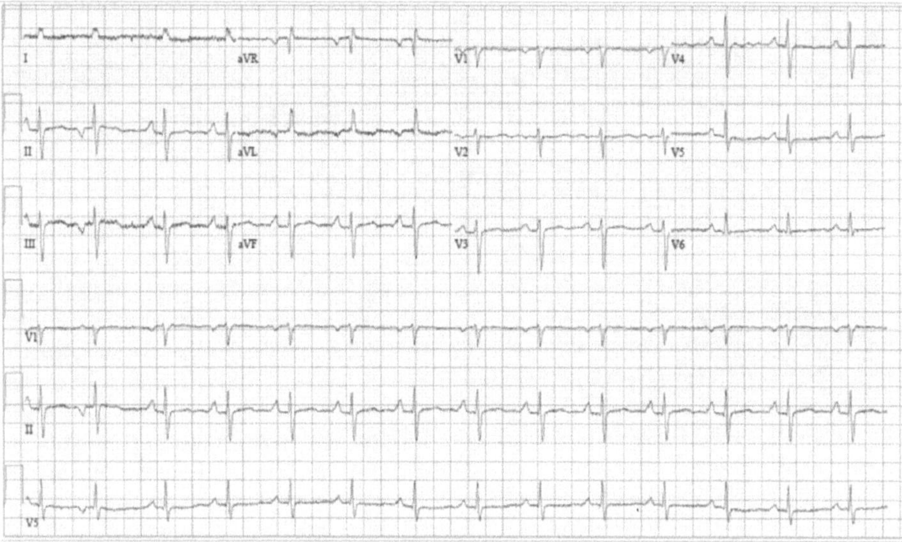

FIGURE 9.18

Rhythm: Sinus rhythm
Rate: 80 BPM
Axis: Right axis deviation (RAD)
Intervals: Normal
P-wave: Right atrial abnormality (RAA)
QRS Complex: Normal
T-wave: Diffuse T-wave flattening
Infarct: None

This ECG demonstrates normal sinus rhythm (NSR) as the P-waves in Leads I, II, and aVF are positive. The P-wave in Lead II is consistent with "P-pulmonale," insofar as it is >2.5 mm in amplitude; all three of the inferior leads (Leads II, III, and aVF) display a similar morphology. This pattern is consistent with a right atrial abnormality (RAA). Also present is a right axis deviation (RAD), as the S-wave in Lead I is greater in amplitude than the corresponding R-wave, while the QRS complex in Leads II and aVF are positive in amplitude. The 2nd beat on the rhythm strip corresponds to a PAC not originating from the SA node, given its inverted P-wave. There is diffuse T-wave flattening across the precordial and limb Leads.

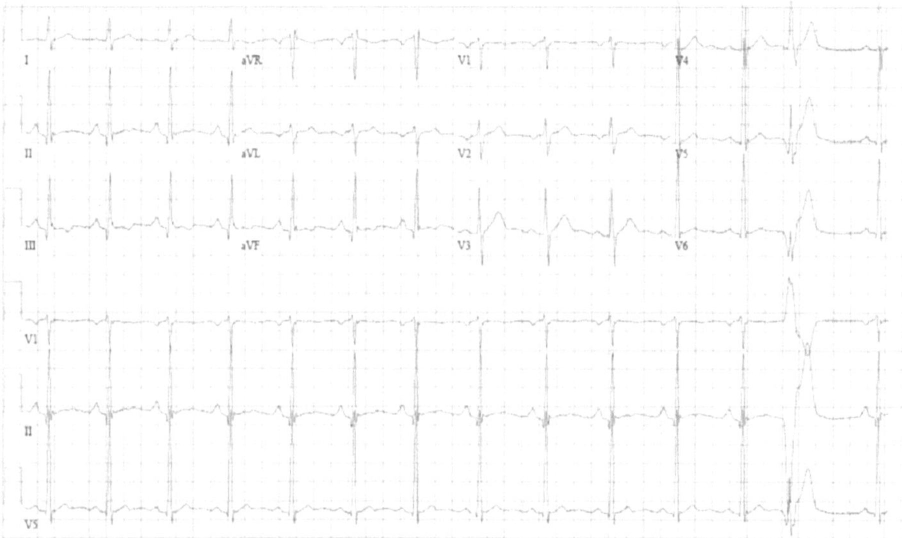

FIGURE 9.19

Rhythm: Sinus rhythm
Rate: 81 BPM
Axis: Normal (Physiologic)
Intervals: ST-segment depressions in Leads III and aVF
P-wave: Biatrial abnormality (BAA)
QRS Complex: Normal
T-wave: T-wave inversions associated with ST-segment depressions in Leads III and aVF
Infarct: None

This ECG demonstrates normal sinus rhythm (NSR) as the P-waves in Leads I, II, and aVF are positive. This tracing represents both a left atrial abnormality (LAA) and a right atrial abnormality (RAA), based upon the P-waves in Leads II, III, and aVF. Namely, the P-waves are ~120 ms in duration and also are ~2.5 mm in amplitude, which correspond to LAA and RAA, respectively. The presence of both LAA and RAA in the same ECG is suggestive of a biatrial abnormality (BAA). A premature ventricular complex (PVC) is best noted as the 13th beat on the rhythm strip; there is a compensatory pause after the PVC depolarizes before the SA node restores normal conduction with another sinus beat. There are T-wave inversions (TWIs) associated with ST-segment depressions in Leads III and aVF.

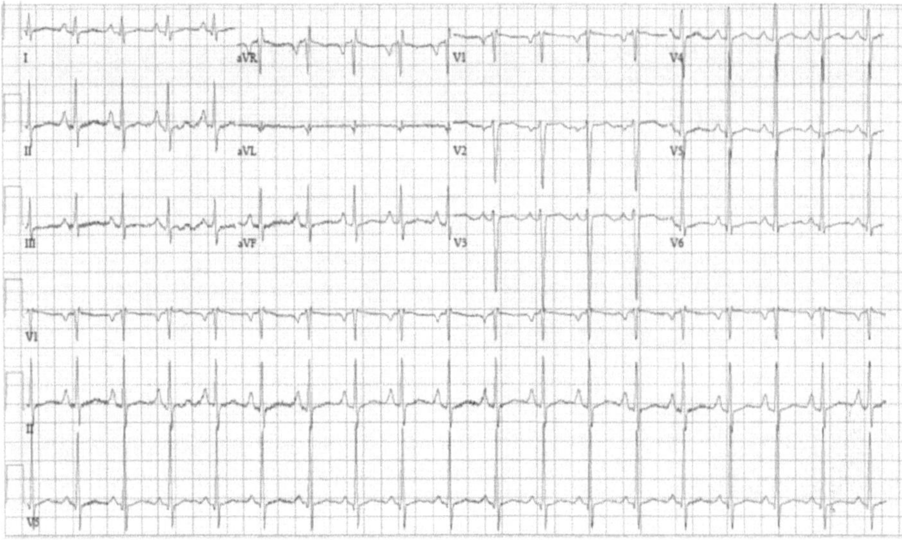

FIGURE 9.20

Rhythm: Sinus tachycardia
Rate: 115 BPM
Axis: Normal (Physiologic)
Intervals: Normal
P-wave: Biatrial abnormality (BAA)
QRS Complex: Normal
T-wave: T-wave flattening in Leads II, III, aVF, V5, and V6
Infarct: None

This ECG demonstrates sinus rhythm as the P-waves in Leads II, III, and aVF are positive. The rate >100 BPM is consistent with tachycardia. This tracing represents both a left atrial abnormality (LAA) and a right atrial abnormality (RAA), based upon the P-waves in Leads II, III, and aVF. Namely, the P-waves are ~120 ms in duration (in addition to the terminal aspect of the P-wave in Lead V1 being ~40 ms in duration and >1 mm deep) and also are ~2.5 mm in amplitude, which correspond to LAA and RAA, respectively. The presence of both LAA and RAA in the same ECG is suggestive of a biatrial abnormality (BAA). There is T-wave flattening in Leads II, III, aVF, V5, and V6.

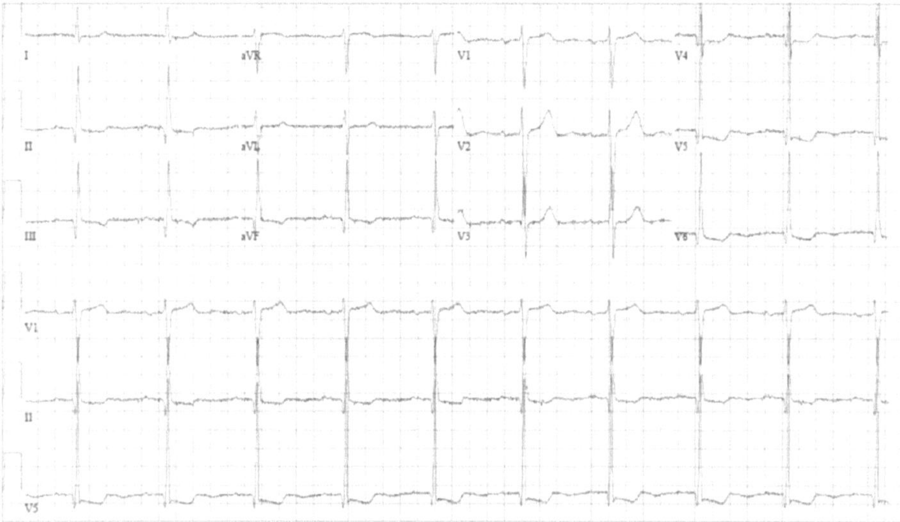

FIGURE 9.21

Rhythm: Sinus rhythm
Rate: 60 BPM
Axis: Normal (Physiologic)
Intervals: PR interval >200 ms (1st Degree AV delay); ST-segment depressions (STDs) in Leads II, III, aVF, and V4–V6
P-wave: Normal
QRS Complex: Left ventricular hypertrophy (LVH)
T-wave: T-wave inversions (TWIs) within Leads II, III, aVF, and V4–V6
Infarct: Prior inferior wall myocardial infarction

This ECG demonstrates sinus rhythm, as the P-waves in Leads I, II, and aVF are positive, and the P-wave in Lead V1 is biphasic. The PR interval is >200 ms, which is indicative of a 1st degree atrioventricular (AV) delay. Note that a 1st degree AV delay is not referred to as an AV block in this text because a QRS is not "dropped," as would be the case with higher-degree blocks. Based upon the Sokolow–Lyon criteria—namely the sum of the mV in V1S and V5R—left ventricular hypertrophy (LVH) is present. There is also evidence of a secondary repolarization abnormality from the LVH, as demonstrated by concave ST-segment depressions (STDs) and associated T-wave inversions (TWIs) within Leads II, III, aVF, and V4–V6. Q-waves in the Leads II, III, and aVF may be indicative of a prior inferior wall myocardial infarction.

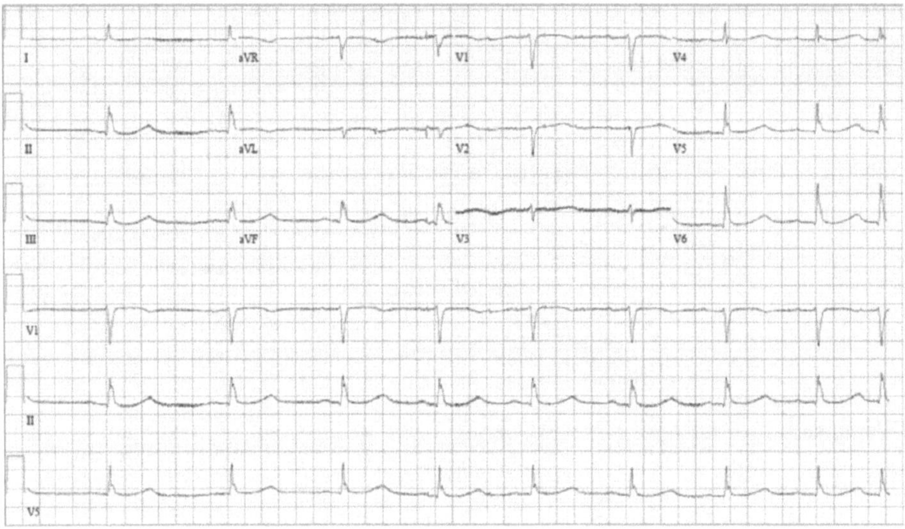

FIGURE 9.22

Rhythm: Sinus bradycardia
Rate: 55 BPM
Axis: Normal (Physiologic)
Intervals: PR interval >200 ms (1st Degree AV delay); QT-interval prolongation >500 ms
P-wave: Normal
QRS Complex: Normal
T-wave: T-wave flattening along Leads I, aVL, and V1–V3
Infarct: None

This ECG demonstrates sinus rhythm, as the P-waves in Leads I, II, and aVF are positive, and the P-wave in Lead V1 is biphasic. The rate <60 BPM is consistent with bradycardia. The PR interval is >200 ms, which is indicative of a 1st degree atrioventricular (AV) delay. Note that a 1st degree AV delay is not referred to as an AV block in this text because a QRS is not "dropped," as would be the case with higher-degree blocks. The corrected QT-interval (QTc) is prolonged in this tracing, being >450 ms in duration. In this particular ECG, the uncorrected QT-interval is in excess of 600 ms. There is T-wave flattening along Leads I, aVL, and V1–V3.

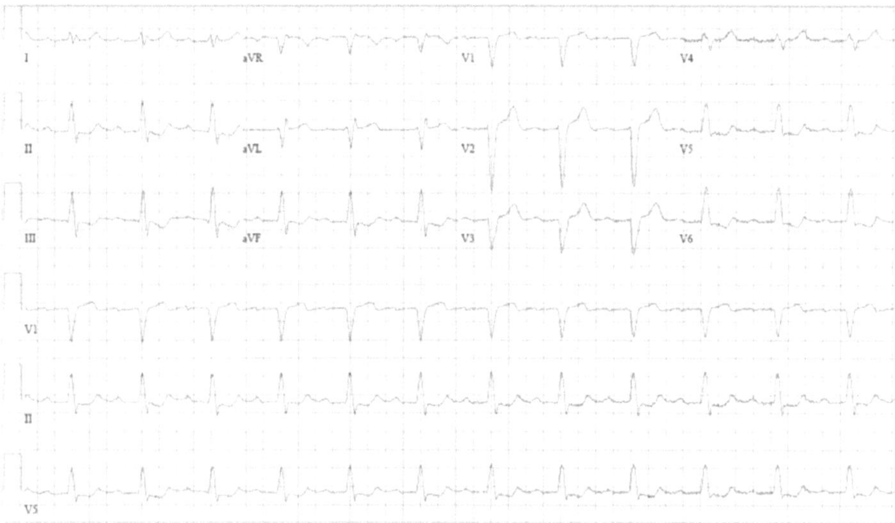

FIGURE 9.23

Rhythm: Sinus rhythm
Rate: 74 BPM
Axis: Normal (Physiologic)
Intervals: ST-segment depressions (STDs) in Leads III, aVF, V5, and V6; PR-interval >200 ms (1st Degree AV delay)
P-wave: Normal
QRS Complex: Left bundle branch block (LBBB)
T-wave: T-wave inversions (TWIs) present in Leads III, aVF, V5, and V6
Infarct: None

This ECG demonstrates sinus rhythm, as the P-waves in Leads I, II, and aVF are positive, and the P-wave in Lead V1 is biphasic. The PR interval is >200 ms, which is indicative of a 1st degree atrioventricular (AV) delay. Note that a 1st degree AV delay is not referred to as an AV block in this text because a QRS is not "dropped," as would be the case with higher-degree blocks. Also present is a left bundle branch block (LBBB) (best appreciated in Leads V1, V2, and V6) with a typical qS-wave in Lead V1, a monophasic R-wave in Lead V6, and a total QRS complex duration of >120 ms. There are ST-segment depressions (STDs) and T-wave inversions (TWIs) in Leads III, aVF, V5, and V6.

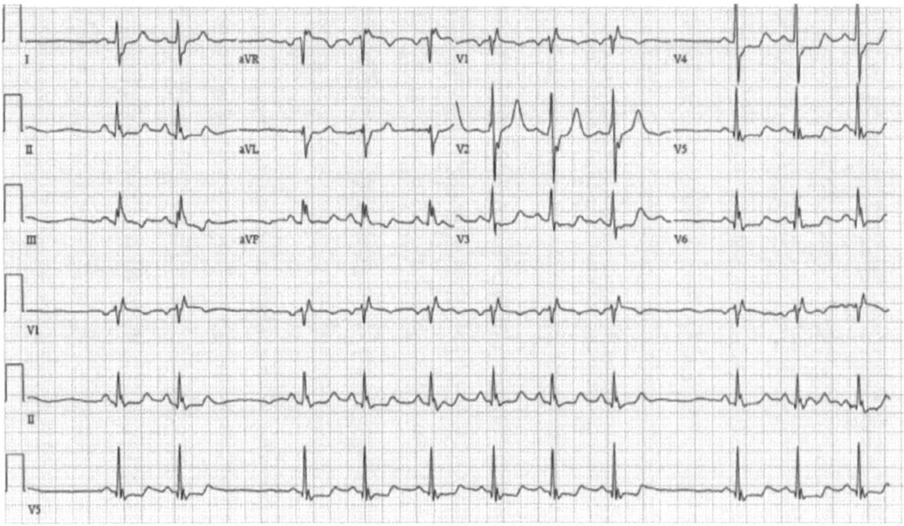

FIGURE 9.24

Rhythm: Sinus rhythm, Sinus exit block
Rate: 66 BPM
Axis: Right axis deviation (RAD)
Intervals: QRS complex duration >200 ms
P-wave: Left atrial abnormality (LAA)
QRS Complex: Right bundle branch block (RBBB); Left posterior hemiblock (LPH); Bifascicular block (BFB)
T-wave: Diffuse ST-segment depressions (STD); T-wave inversions (TWI)
Infarct: None

This ECG demonstrates normal sinus rhythm (NSR), as the P-waves in Leads I, II, and aVF are positive, and the P-wave in Lead V1 is biphasic. There is a sinus exit block present, as a pause occurs after the 2nd and 8th beats on the rhythm strip. The duration of the exit block is double the PP-interval of the antecedent beats, and the PR-segment of these same beats does not appear to prolong. As such, this tracing is reflective of sinoatrial (SA) Mobitz Type II. An rSR' is present in Lead V1, and the QRS complex is >120 ms in duration, which is consistent with a right bundle branch block (RBBB). Furthermore, a right axis deviation (RAD) is present, as the S-wave in Lead I is greater in amplitude than the corresponding R-wave, while the QRS complex in Leads II and aVF are positive in amplitude. Additionally, there is an rS-wave present in Leads I and aVL, a qR-wave in Lead III, and a QRS complex that is between 80 ms and 100 ms in duration. This pattern is demonstrative of a left posterior fascicular block (LPFB), which is also known as a left posterior hemiblock (LPH). Collectively, the presence of an RBBB and an LAH in the same ECG is diagnostic for a bifascicular block (BFB). The deep terminal aspect of the P-wave in Lead V1 and P-wave >120 ms in Lead II points to an LAA as well.

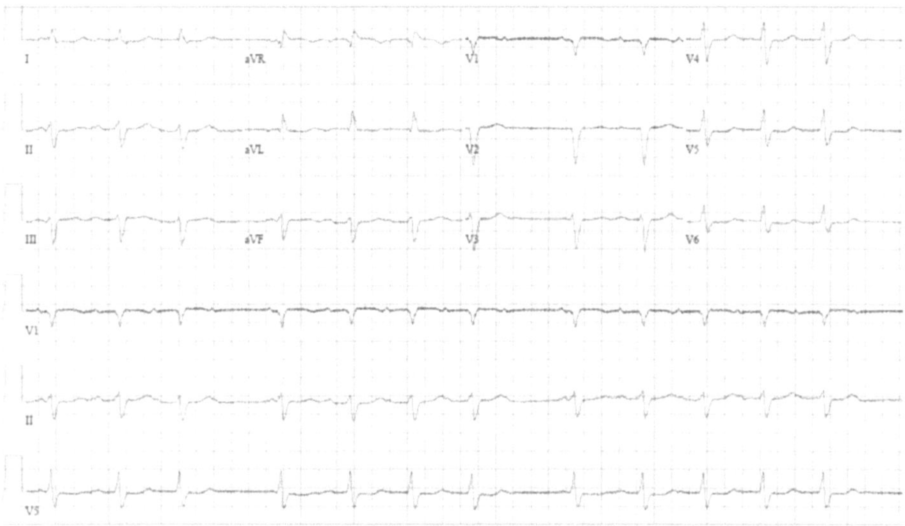

FIGURE 9.25

Rhythm: Sinus rhythm with 2nd Degree AV block, Mobitz Type I
Rate: 72 BPM
Axis: Left axis deviation (LAD)
Intervals: Progressively prolonging PR-interval with QRS dropping
P-wave: Normal
QRS Complex: Intraventricular conduction delay (IVCD)
T-wave: T-wave flattening in Leads III, aVF, aVL, and V1–V3
Infarct: Prior septal myocardial infarction

This ECG demonstrates sinus rhythm, as the P-waves in Leads I, II, and aVF are positive. However, the PR segment becomes progressively longer until a P-wave is not conducted, and a QRS complex is "dropped." Progressive PR-interval prolongation is evident on the 1st, 2nd, and 3rd beats of the rhythm strip, with the 4th P-wave not being associated with a QRS complex. There is a concomitant shortening of the RR-interval in the aforementioned beats as well. This pattern is consistent with 2nd degree atrioventricular block (AVB), Mobitz Type I (also known as Wenckebach), and can be seen continually on the rhythm strip. The RR-interval that contains the non-conducted P-wave is <2 times the PP-intervals in duration. There is a nonspecific intraventricular conduction delay (IVCD), which is seen with a QRS complex duration of >110 ms in the absence of full morphological criteria for a left or right bundle branch block (LBBB/RBBB). Additionally, there is a left axis deviation (LAD) present in this ECG, as indicated by the R-wave amplitude > S-wave amplitude in Lead I, in contrast to the R-wave amplitude < S-wave amplitude in Lead II. There is T-wave flattening in Leads III, aVF, aVL, and V1–V3. Q-waves in Leads V1 and V2 are concerning for a prior septal myocardial infarction.

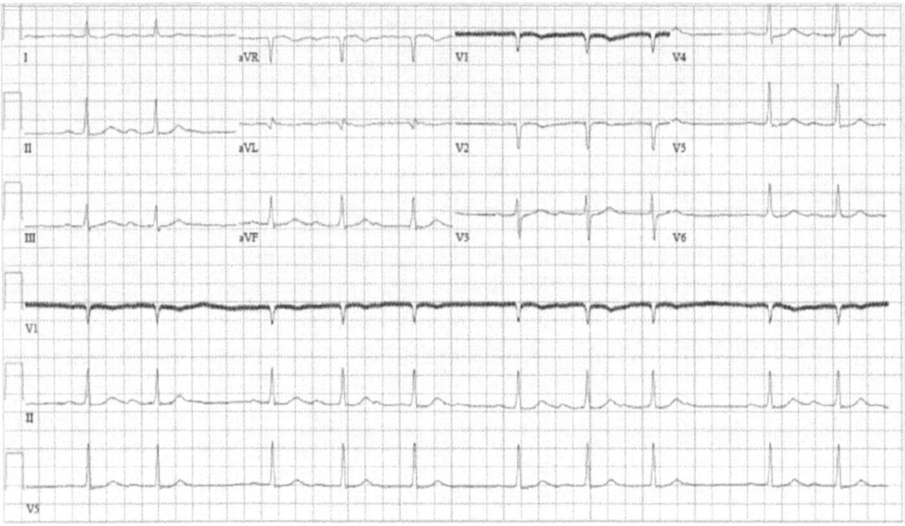

FIGURE 9.26

Rhythm: Sinus rhythm with 2nd Degree AV block, Mobitz Type I
Rate: 60 BPM
Axis: Normal (Physiologic)
Intervals: Progressively prolonging PR-interval with QRS dropping
P-wave: Normal
QRS Complex: Normal
T-wave: Normal
Infarct: None

This ECG demonstrates sinus rhythm, as the P-waves in Leads I, II, and aVF are positive. However, the PR segment becomes progressively longer until a P-wave is not conducted, and a QRS complex is "dropped." Progressive PR-interval prolongation is evident throughout the tracing. Specifically, a pattern known as "group beating" can be seen; the 1st and 2nd beats are grouped together, as are the 3rd through 5th beats, and the 6th through 8th beats. The RR-interval that contains the non-conducted P-wave is <2 times the PP-intervals in duration. This pattern can also be seen with 2nd degree atrioventricular block (AVB), Mobitz Type I (also known as Wenckebach), and can be seen continually on the rhythm strip. Incidentally, an artifact is present along Lead V1, causing a thickening of the line. This is likely in the context of myopotentials from skeletal muscles that lie adjacent to the aforementioned Lead and could also represent an issue with ECG machine itself.

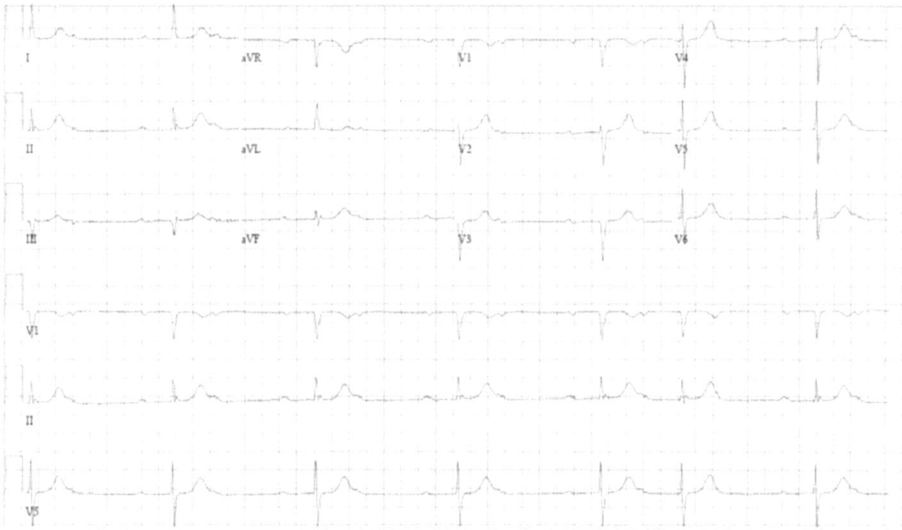

FIGURE 9.27

Rhythm: Sinus bradycardia with 2:1 AV block, 2nd Degree AV block, Mobitz Type I
Rate: 40 BPM
Axis: Normal (Physiologic)
Intervals: PR-interval >200 ms (1st Degree AV delay)
P-wave: Normal
QRS Complex: Poor R-wave progression (PRWP)
T-wave: Normal
Infarct: None

This ECG demonstrates sinus rhythm, as the P-waves in Leads I, II, and aVF are positive. The rate <60 BPM is consistent with bradycardia. However, every other P-wave in this tracing is non-conducted, resulting in a dropped QRS complex. As such, there is a fixed ratio of two P-waves for every QRS complex—this morphology is referred to as 2:1 atrioventricular block (2:1 AVB). The PR interval is >200 ms, which is indicative of a 1st degree atrioventricular (AV) delay. Because it is not feasible to determine if any changes to the PR-interval occur prior to the dropped QRS complex, the terms "Mobitz" and "Wenckebach" are not used in this context. However, the last few beats due conduct in a row with a prolonging PR-interval, indicative of unmasked 2nd degree AV block, Mobitz Type I.

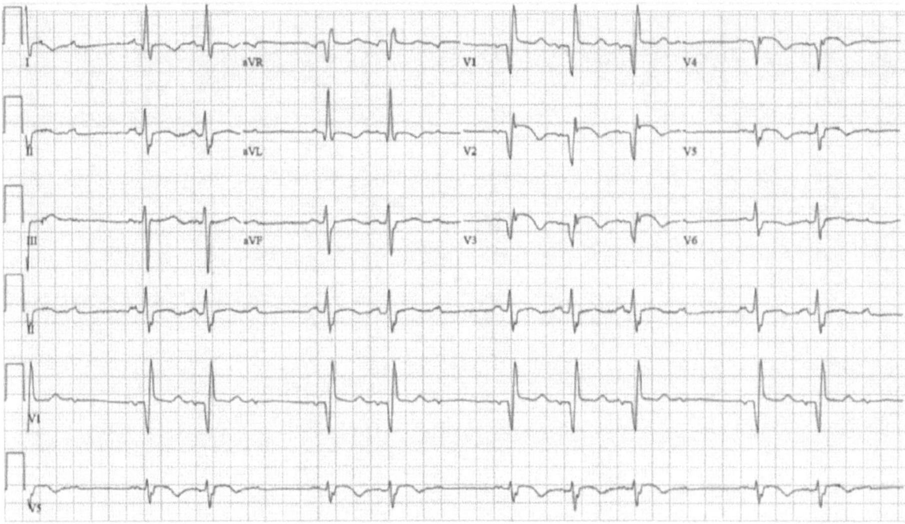

FIGURE 9.28

Rhythm: Sinus bradycardia with 2nd Degree AV block, Mobitz Type II
Rate: 58 BPM
Axis: Normal (Physiologic)
Intervals: Normal
P-wave: Normal
QRS Complex: Poor R-wave progression (PRWP); Right bundle branch block (RBBB)
T-wave: T-wave inversions (TWIs) in leads I, aVL, II, and V2–V6
Infarct: Prior anteroseptal myocardial infarction

This ECG demonstrates sinus rhythm, as the P-waves in Leads I, II, and aVF are positive. However, after the 1st, 3rd, 5th, 8th, and 10th beats on the rhythm strip, there are P-waves that are not conducted to a QRS complex. While these P-waves are non-conducted, leading to a "dropped" QRS complex, there is no antecedent PR-interval prolongation, nor is there a concomitant shortening of the RR-interval. Group beating is present in this tracing, comprised of the 2nd and 3rd beats, as well as beats 4 and 5, beats 6 through 8, and beats 9 and 10. The RR-interval containing the non-conducted P-wave is equivalent in duration to double the PP-interval. This suggests the presence of 2nd degree atrioventricular block (AVB), Mobitz Type II. Poor R-wave progression (PRWP) is present along the precordial leads, as the QRS complex does not become positive (aside from Lead V1) until Lead V6, with the isoelectric point between Leads V5 and V6. An rSR' is present in Lead V1, and the QRS complex is >120 ms in duration, which is consistent with a right bundle branch block (RBBB). There are T-wave inversions (TWIs) in leads I, aVL, II, and V2–V6. Q-waves present in Leads V1–V4 raise concern for a prior anteroseptal myocardial infarction.

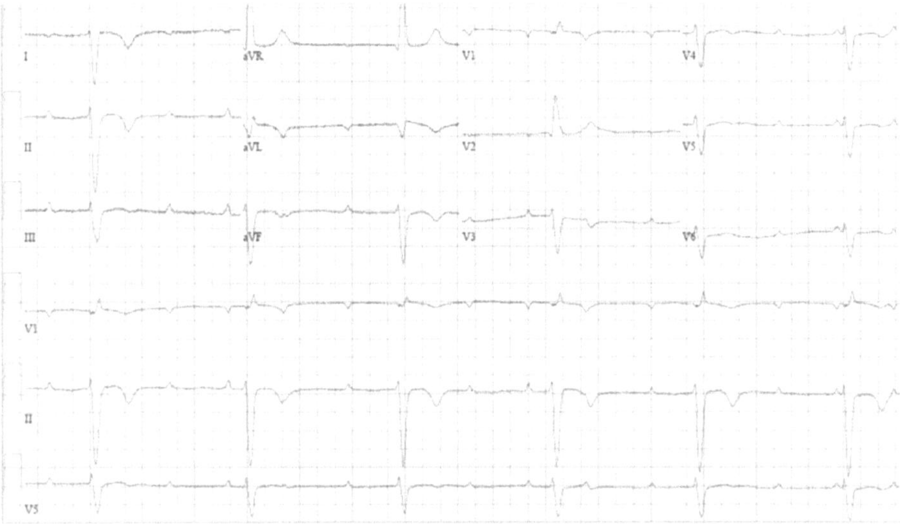

FIGURE 9.29

Rhythm: Sinus rhythm with 3rd Degree AV block (CHB)
Rate: 34 BPM
Axis: Northwestern axis deviation
Intervals: Constant PP and RR intervals
P-wave: Normal
QRS Complex: Sinus rhythm with 3rd Degree AV block (CHB)
T-wave: Not applicable with ventricular escape rhythm
Infarct: Prior septal myocardial infarction

This ECG demonstrates a possible ectopic atrial rhythm, given the negative amplitude of the P-waves in Leads I and V1, despite positive deflections in Leads II and aVF. Moreover, there are P-waves throughout the rhythm strip that do not conduct to an associated QRS complex. However, the PP-interval and RR-interval remain constant throughout the tracing, while the PR-interval varies. The atrial rate (around 90 BPM) is faster than the ventricular rate (around 35 BPM); the atria and the ventricles are depolarizing independently of one another. This pattern of AV dissociation in the context of an atrial rate faster than the ventricular rate is consistent with 3rd degree atrioventricular block (AVB), otherwise known as complete heart block (CHB). This CHB has a wide escape rhythm, as indicated by the QRS complex duration >120 ms. The QRS axis on this tracing is a Northwestern axis (also known as an extreme right axis, or a superior axis), due to the S-waves in both Leads I and II being greater in amplitude than their respective R-waves. Alternatively, the Northwestern axis may be due to right arm and left arm lead switch due to the positive QRS complex polarity in Lead aVR and negative QRS complex polarity in Lead aVL. Q-waves present in Leads V1 and V2 raise concern for a prior septal myocardial infarction.

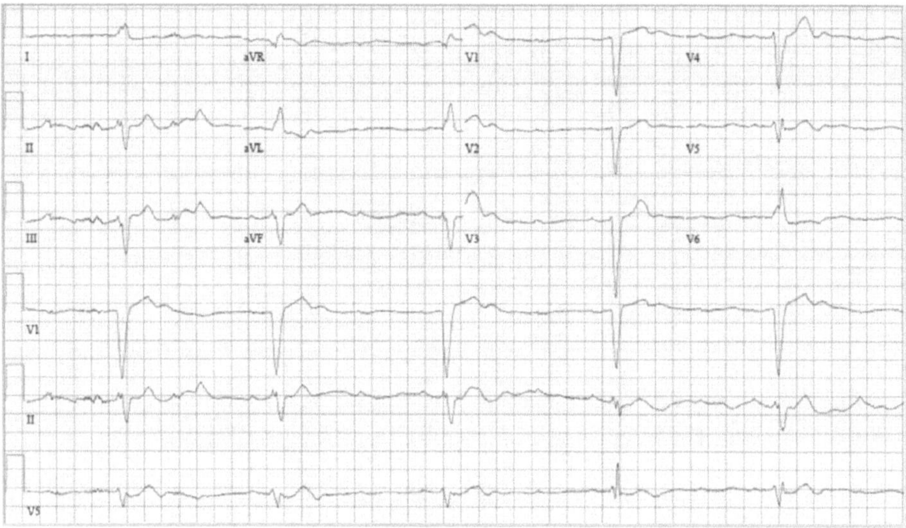

FIGURE 9.30

Rhythm: Sinus rhythm with 3rd Degree AV block (CHB)
Rate: 32 BPM
Axis: Left axis deviation (LAD)
Intervals: Constant PP and RR intervals
P-wave: Normal
QRS Complex: Wide ventricular escape
T-wave: Not applicable with ventricular escape rhythm
Infarct: None

This ECG demonstrates sinus rhythm, as the P-waves in Leads I, II, and aVF are positive. There are P-waves that are evident throughout the rhythm strip that do not conduct to an associated QRS complex. However, the PP-interval and RR-interval remain constant throughout the tracing, while the PR-interval varies. The atrial rate (around 80 BPM) is faster than the ventricular rate (around 30 BPM); the atria and the ventricles are depolarizing independently of one another. This pattern of AV dissociation in the context of an atrial rate faster than the ventricular rate is consistent with 3rd degree atrioventricular block (AVB), otherwise known as complete heart block (CHB). This CHB has a wide escape rhythm, as indicated by the QRS complex duration >120 ms. There is a left axis deviation (LAD) present in this ECG as well, as indicated by the R-wave amplitude > S-wave amplitude in Lead I, in contrast to the R-wave amplitude < S-wave amplitude in Lead II.

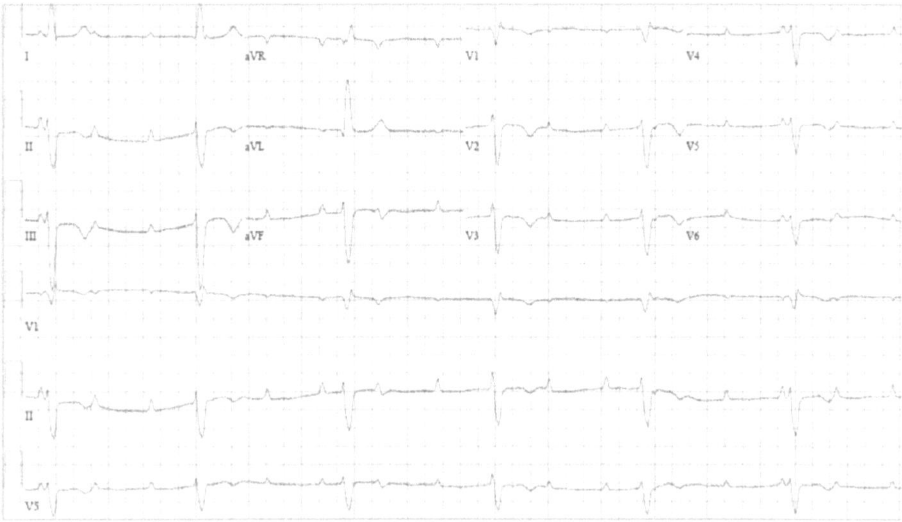

FIGURE 9.31

Rhythm: Sinus rhythm with 3rd Degree AV block (CHB)
Rate: 36 BPM
Axis: Left axis deviation (LAD)
Intervals: Constant PP and RR intervals
P-wave: Right atrial abnormality (RAA)
QRS Complex: Wide wscape rhythm
T-wave: Not applicable with ventricular escape rhythm
Infarct: None

This ECG demonstrates sinus rhythm, as the P-waves in Leads I, II, and aVF are positive. There are P-waves that are evident throughout the rhythm strip that do not conduct to an associated QRS complex. However, the PP-interval and RR-interval remain constant throughout the tracing, while the PR-interval varies. The atrial rate (around 100 BPM) is faster than the ventricular rate (around 35 BPM); the atria and the ventricles are depolarizing independently of one another. This pattern of AV dissociation in the context of an atrial rate faster than the ventricular rate is consistent with 3rd degree atrioventricular block (AVB), otherwise known as complete heart block (CHB). This CHB has a wide escape rhythm, as indicated by the QRS complex duration >120 ms. There is a left axis deviation (LAD) present in this ECG as well, as indicated by the R-wave amplitude > S-wave amplitude in Lead I, in contrast to the R-wave amplitude < S-wave amplitude in Lead II. The P-wave in Lead II is consistent with "P-pulmonale," insofar as it is >2.5 mm in amplitude; all three of the inferior leads (Leads II, III, and aVF) display a similar morphology. This pattern is consistent with a right atrial abnormality (RAA).

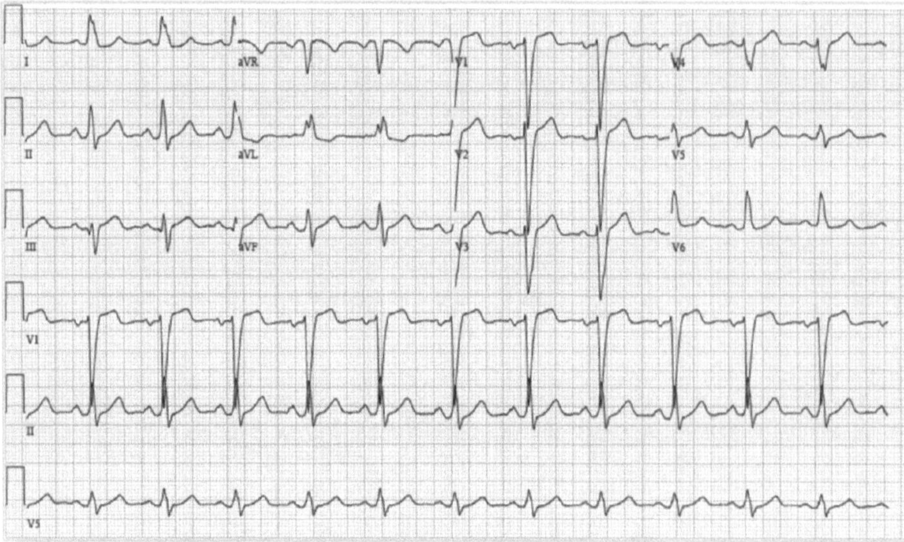

FIGURE 9.32

Rhythm: Sinus rhythm
Rate: 74 BPM
Axis: Normal (Physiologic)
Intervals: QRS complex duration >120 ms
P-wave: Borderline left atrial abnormality (LAA)
QRS Complex: Left bundle branch block (LBBB)
T-wave: Repolarization abnormalities from LBBB
Infarct: None

This ECG demonstrates normal sinus rhythm (NSR), as the P-waves in Leads I, II, and aVF are positive, and the P-wave in Lead V1 is biphasic. Also present is a left bundle branch block (LBBB) (best appreciated in Leads V1, V2, and V6) with a typical rS-wave in Lead V1, a monophasic R-wave in Lead V6, and a total QRS complex duration of >120 ms. There is also notching in the R-waves of Leads I and aVL from the LBBB. Due to the terminal component of the biphasic P-wave in Lead V1, being ~1 small box deep and wide (~1 mm deep and ~40 ms wide), there is a possible left atrial abnormality (LAA) present.

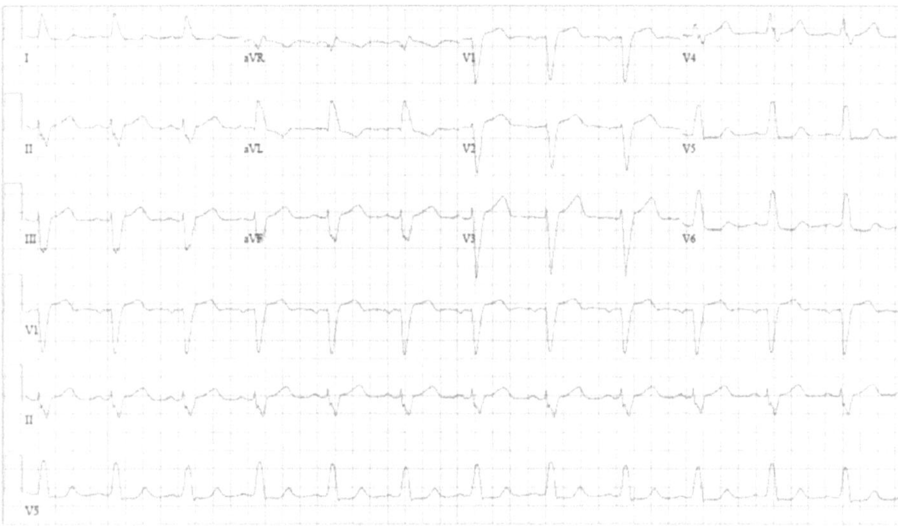

FIGURE 9.33

Rhythm: Sinus rhythm
Rate: 72 BPM
Axis: Left axis deviation (LAD)
Intervals: ST-segment depressions (STDs) in Leads I, V5, and V6
P-wave: Normal
QRS Complex: Left bundle branch block (LBBB)
T-wave: T-wave inversion (TWI) in Lead aVL
Infarct: None

This ECG demonstrates sinus rhythm, as the P-waves in Leads I, II, and aVF are positive, and the P-wave in Lead V1 is biphasic. Also present is a left bundle branch block (LBBB) (best appreciated in Leads V1, V2, and V6) with a typical QS-wave in Lead V1, a monophasic R-wave in Lead V6, and a total QRS complex duration of >120 ms. Additionally, there is at least a 50 ms delay in the onset of the intrinsicoid deflection (beginning of the QRS complex to the peak of the R-wave) in Leads I, V5, and V6. There is a notable "notching" of the QRS complex in the aforementioned Leads, along with discordant ST-segment changes (ST-segment elevations in Leads V1–V3, ST-segment depressions in Leads I, V5, and V6). There is a left axis deviation (LAD) present in this ECG as well, as indicated by the R-wave amplitude > S-wave amplitude in Lead I, in contrast to the R-wave amplitude < S-wave amplitude in Lead II. There is a T-wave inversion (TWI) in Lead aVL.

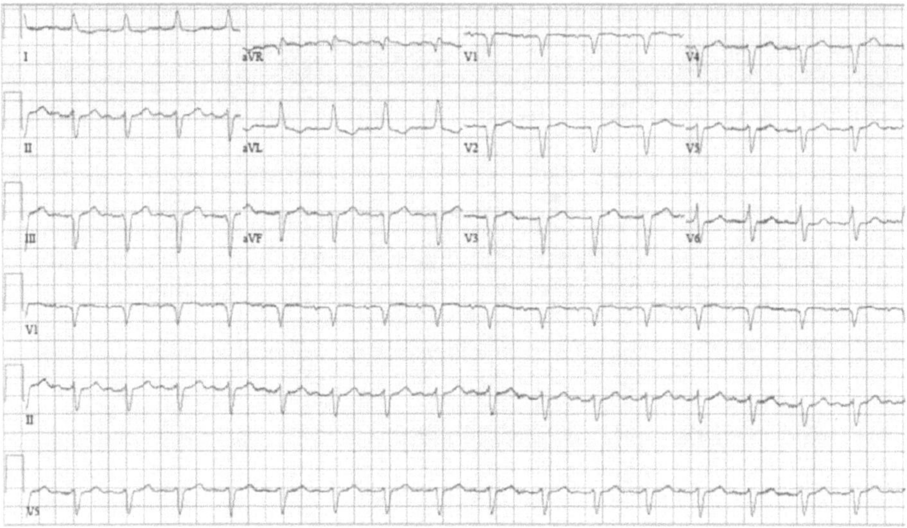

FIGURE 9.34

Rhythm: Sinus tachycardia
Rate: 102 BPM
Axis: Left axis deviation (LAD)
Intervals: PR-interval >200 ms (1st Degree AV delay)
P-wave: Normal
QRS Complex: Left bundle branch block (LBBB)
T-wave: T-wave inversions (TWIs) in Leads I, aVL, V5, and V6
Infarct: Prior anteroseptal myocardial infarction

This ECG demonstrates sinus rhythm as the P-waves in Leads I, II, and aVF are positive, and the P-wave in Lead V1 is biphasic. The rate >100 BPM is consistent with tachycardia. Also present is a left bundle branch block (LBBB) (best appreciated in Leads V1, V2, and V6) with a typical QS-wave in Lead V1, and a total QRS complex duration of >120 ms. Additionally, there is at least a 50 ms delay in the onset of the intrinsicoid deflection (beginning of the QRS complex to the peak of the R-wave) in Leads I, V5, and V6. There is a notable "notching" of the QRS complex in the aforementioned Leads, along with discordant ST-segment changes (ST-segment elevations in Leads V1–V3, ST-segment depressions and T-wave inversions in Leads I, aVL, V5, and V6). The presence of QS-waves in contiguous Leads (specifically, Leads V1 and V2) raises the possibility of an anteroseptal myocardial infarction of unknown age. There is a left axis deviation (LAD) present in this ECG as well, as indicated by the R-wave amplitude > S-wave amplitude in Lead I, in contrast to the R-wave amplitude < S-wave amplitude in Lead II. The PR interval is >200 ms, which is indicative of a 1st degree atrioventricular (AV) delay.

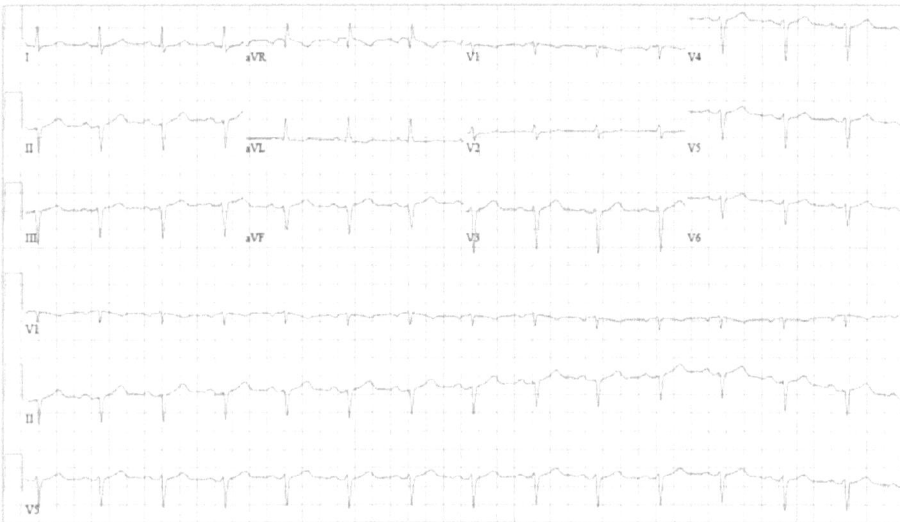

FIGURE 9.35

Rhythm: Sinus rhythm
Rate: 87 BPM
Axis: Left axis deviation (LAD)
Intervals: Normal
P-wave: Normal
QRS Complex: Left anterior hemiblock (LAH); Poor R-wave progression (PRWP)
T-wave: Normal
Infarct: None

This ECG demonstrates sinus rhythm as the P-waves in Leads I, II, and aVF are positive. There is a left axis deviation (LAD) present in this ECG as well, as indicated by the R-wave amplitude > S-wave amplitude in Lead I, in contrast to the R-wave amplitude < S-wave amplitude in Lead II. Additionally, there is a qR-wave present in Leads I and aVL, an rS-wave in Lead III, and a QRS complex that is between 80 ms and 100 ms in duration. This pattern is demonstrative of a left anterior fascicular block (LAFB), which is also known as a left anterior hemiblock (LAH). This occurs when the anterior fascicle of the left bundle branch is lesioned, causing conduction down that fascicle to be delayed. Other etiologies of LAD, such as LVH, inferior wall myocardial infarction (MI), complete LBBB, obstructive lung disease, and congenital heart disease, must be ruled out before the diagnosis of LAH can be made. There is an associated poor R-wave progression (PRWP) along the precordial leads, as the QRS complex does not become positive throughout the precordial leads, aside from Lead V2, with Leads V3–V6 remaining negative.

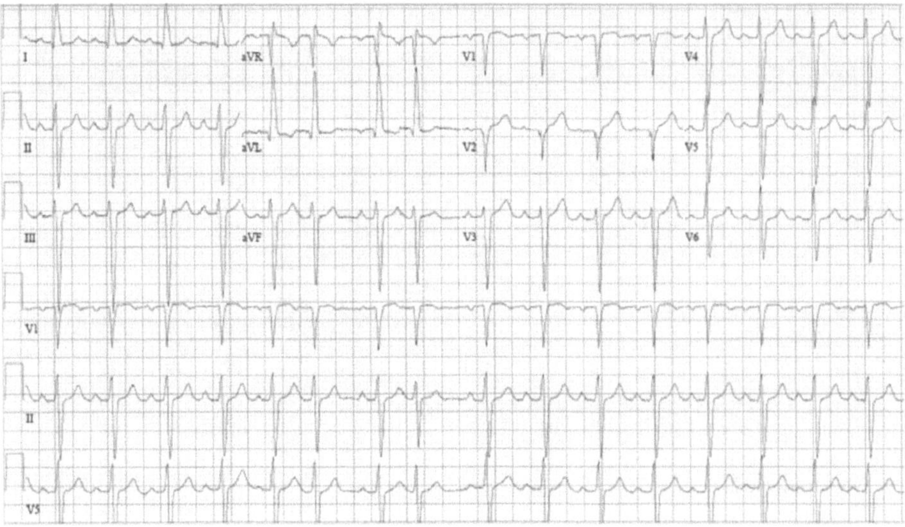

FIGURE 9.36

Rhythm: Sinus rhythm
Rate: 95 BPM
Axis: Left axis deviation (LAD)
Intervals: Normal
P-wave: Normal
QRS Complex: Left anterior hemiblock (LAH); Poor R-wave progression (PRWP)
T-wave: Normal
Infarct: None

This ECG demonstrates sinus rhythm as the P-waves in Leads I, II, and aVF are positive, the P-wave in Lead V1 is biphasic. There is a left axis deviation (LAD) present in this ECG as well, as indicated by the R-wave amplitude > S-wave amplitude in Lead I, in contrast to the R-wave amplitude < S-wave amplitude in Lead II. Additionally, there is a qR-wave present in Leads I and aVL, an rS-wave in Lead III, and a QRS complex that is between 80 ms and 100 ms in duration. This pattern is demonstrative of a left anterior fascicular block (LAFB), which is also known as a left anterior hemiblock (LAH). This occurs when the anterior fascicle of the left bundle branch is lesioned, causing conduction down that fascicle to be delayed. Other etiologies of LAD, such as LVH, inferior wall myocardial infarction (MI), complete LBBB, and obstructive lung disease, and congenital heart disease must be ruled out before the diagnosis of LAH can be made. The PR interval is >200 ms, which is indicative of a 1st degree atrioventricular (AV) delay. The 6th and 8th beats on the rhythm strip correspond to premature atrial contractions (PACs) and are followed by a compensatory pause in both instances. There is an associated poor R-wave progression (PRWP) along the precordial leads, as the QRS complex does not become positive by Lead V6.

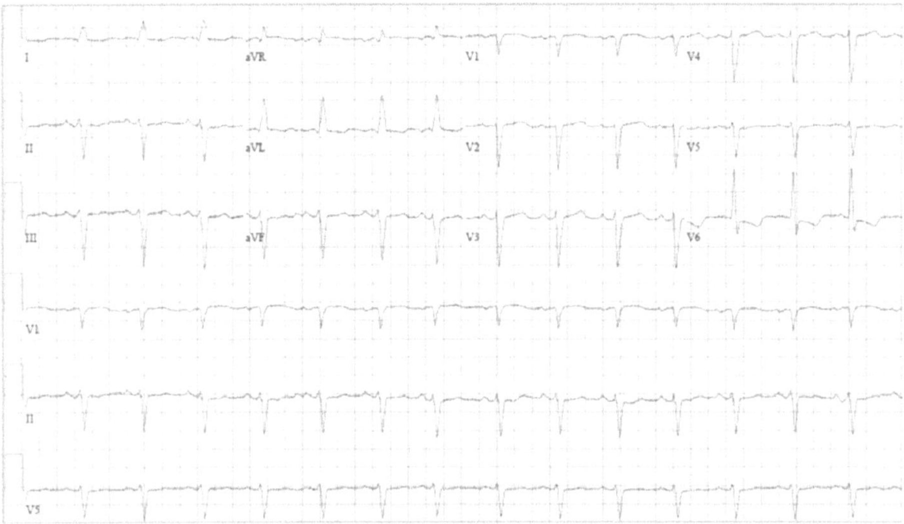

FIGURE 9.37

Rhythm: Sinus rhythm
Rate: 91 BPM
Axis: Left axis deviation (LAD)
Intervals: ST-segment depressions in Leads I, aVL, and V6
P-wave: Normal
QRS Complex: Left anterior hemiblock (LAH); Poor R-wave progression (PRWP)
T-wave: T-wave inversions in Leads I, aVL, and V6
Infarct: None

This ECG demonstrates sinus rhythm as the P-waves in Leads I, II, and aVF are positive, the P-wave in Lead V1 is biphasic. There is a left axis deviation (LAD) present in this ECG as well, as indicated by the R-wave amplitude > S-wave amplitude in Lead I, in contrast to the R-wave amplitude < S-wave amplitude in Lead II. Additionally, there is a qR-wave present in Leads I and aVL, an rS-wave in Lead III, and a QRS complex that is between 80 ms and 100 ms in duration. This pattern is demonstrative of a left anterior fascicular block (LAFB), which is also known as a left anterior hemiblock (LAH). This occurs when the anterior fascicle of the left bundle branch is lesioned, causing conduction down that fascicle to be delayed. Other etiologies of LAD, such as LVH, inferior wall myocardial infarction (MI), complete LBBB, and obstructive lung disease, and congenital heart disease must be ruled out before the diagnosis of LAH can be made. There are T-wave inversions and ST-segment depressions in Leads I, aVL, and V6, with T-wave flattening in Lead V5, concerning for lateral ischemia. There is an associated poor R-wave progression (PRWP) along the precordial leads, as the QRS complex does not become positive until Lead V6, with the isoelectric point between Leads V5 and V6.

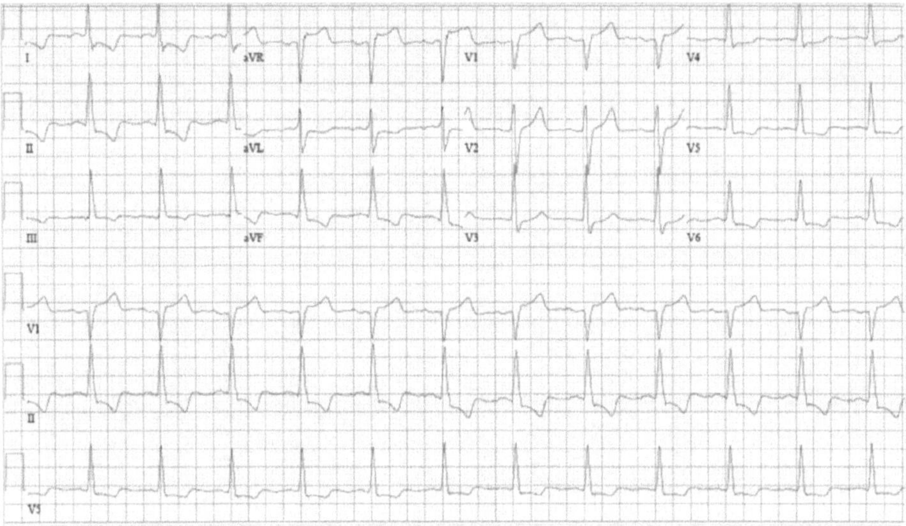

FIGURE 9.38

Rhythm: Sinus rhythm
Rate: 75 BPM
Axis: Normal (Physiologic)
Intervals: ST-segment depressions (STDs) in Leads I, aVL, V5, V6, II, III, and aVF
P-wave: Normal
QRS Complex: Intraventricular Conduction Delay (IVCD)
T-wave: T-wave inversions (TWIs) in Leads I, aVL, V5, V6, II, III, and aVF
Infarct: None

This ECG demonstrates sinus rhythm as the P-waves in Leads I, II, and aVF are positive. A nonspecific intraventricular conduction delay (IVCD) is present, in which the QRS complex is >110 ms in duration (or alternatively, there is a notching of the QRS complex without associated prolongation), but neither a left bundle branch block nor a right bundle branch block (RBBB) morphology is present. There are 2–3 mm ST-segment depressions (STDs) and T-wave inversions (TWIs) in Leads I, aVL, V5, V6, II, III, and aVF, concerning for inferolateral ischemia.

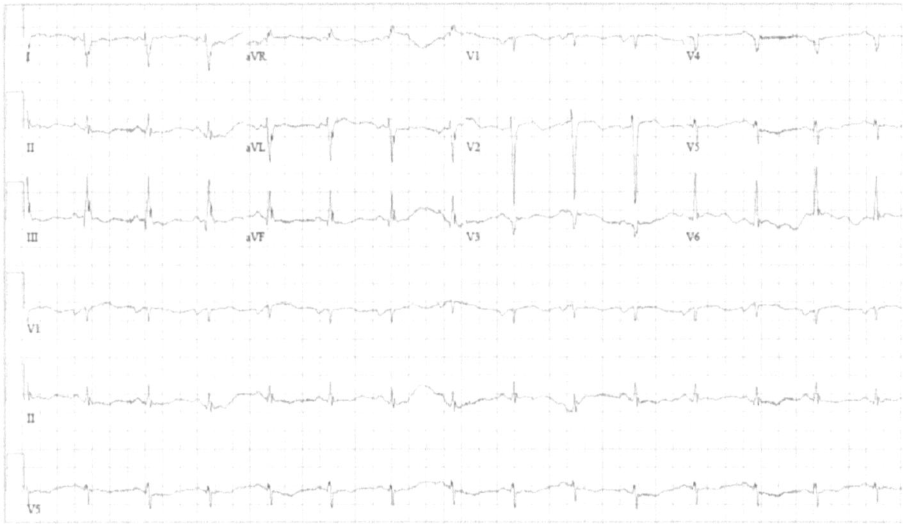

FIGURE 9.39

Rhythm: Sinus rhythm
Rate: 87 BPM
Axis: Right axis deviation (RAD)
Intervals: Normal
P-wave: Normal
QRS Complex: Left posterior hemiblock (LPH); Poor R-wave progression (PRWP)
T-wave: T-wave inversions (TWIs) in Leads II, III, aVF, V5, and V6
Infarct: None

This ECG demonstrates sinus rhythm as the P-waves in Leads I, II, and aVF are positive, the P-wave in Lead V1 is biphasic. A right axis deviation (RAD) is present, as the S-wave in Lead I is greater in amplitude than the corresponding R-wave, while the QRS complex in Leads II and aVF are positive in amplitude. Additionally, there is an rS-wave present in Leads I and aVL, a qR-wave in Lead III, and a QRS complex that is between 80 ms and 100 ms in duration. This pattern is demonstrative of a left posterior fascicular block (LPFB), which is also known as a left posterior hemiblock (LPH). There is an associated poor R-wave progression (PRWP) along the precordial leads, as the QRS complex does not become positive within the precordial leads until Lead V6, aside from Lead V2, with Leads V3–V5 remaining negative. There are T-wave inversions (TWIs) in Leads II, III, aVF, V5, and V6.

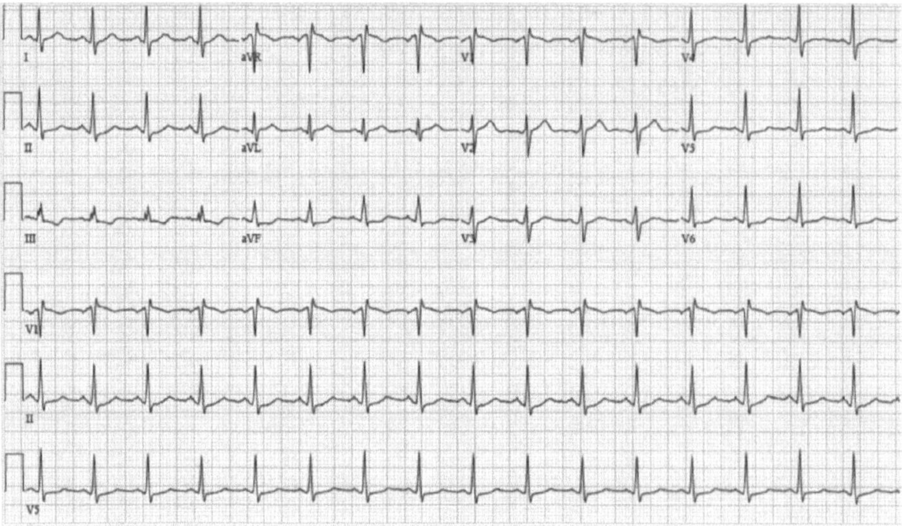

FIGURE 9.40

Rhythm: Sinus rhythm
Rate: 97 BPM
Axis: Normal (Physiologic)
Intervals: Normal
P-wave: Normal
QRS Complex: Incomplete right bundle branch block (iRBBB)
T-wave: T-wave inversion (TWI), T-wave flattening and ST-segment depressions in Lead III and V4–V6.
Infarct: None

This ECG demonstrates sinus rhythm as the P-waves in Leads I, II, and aVF are positive. An rSR' morphology is present in Lead V1 in conjunction with a QRS complex between 100 ms and 120 ms in duration. This is indicative of an incomplete right bundle branch block (incomplete RBBB). There is a T-wave inversion (TWI) in Lead III, along with T-wave flattening in Leads V4–V6. Furthermore, there are ST-segment depressions in the same leads.

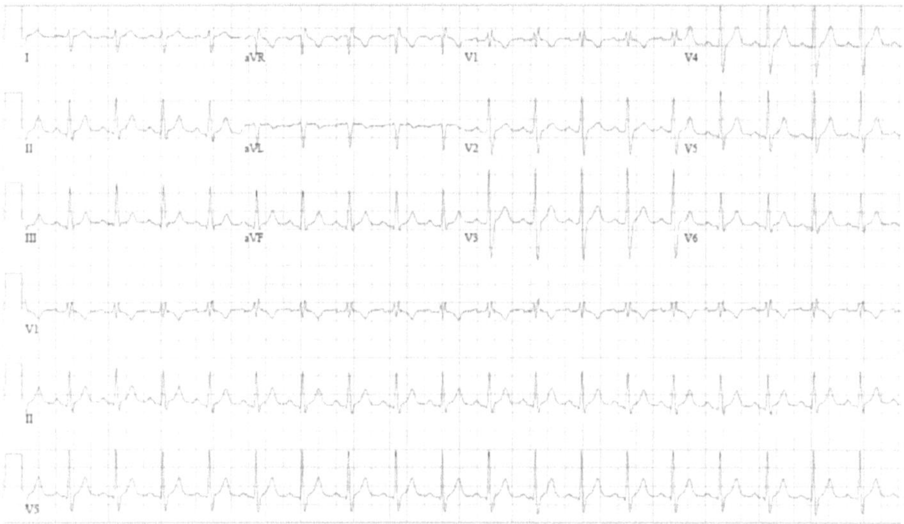

FIGURE 9.41

Rhythm: Sinus tachycardia
Rate: 115 BPM
Axis: Right axis deviation (RAD)
Intervals: Normal
P-wave: Normal
QRS Complex: Left posterior hemiblock (LPH); Incomplete right bundle branch block (iRBBB)
T-wave: Normal
Infarct: None

This ECG demonstrates sinus rhythm as the P-waves in Leads I, II, and aVF are positive, the P-wave in Lead V1 is biphasic. The rate >100 BPM is consistent with tachycardia. A right axis deviation (RAD) is present, as the S-wave in Lead I is greater in amplitude than the corresponding R-wave, while the QRS complex in Leads II and aVF are positive in amplitude. Additionally, there is an rS-wave present in Leads I and aVL, a qR-wave in Lead III, and a QRS complex that is between 80 ms and 100 ms in duration. This pattern is demonstrative of a left posterior fascicular block (LPFB), which is also known as a left posterior hemiblock (LPH). This tracing demonstrates an rSR' morphology in Leads V1 and V2, and is similar in morphology to a complete right bundle branch block (RBBB). However, the QRS complex duration is between 90 ms and 120 ms in duration, rather than the >120 ms that would be diagnostic for a complete RBBB. As such, this tracing is most consistent with an incomplete RBBB (iRBBB).

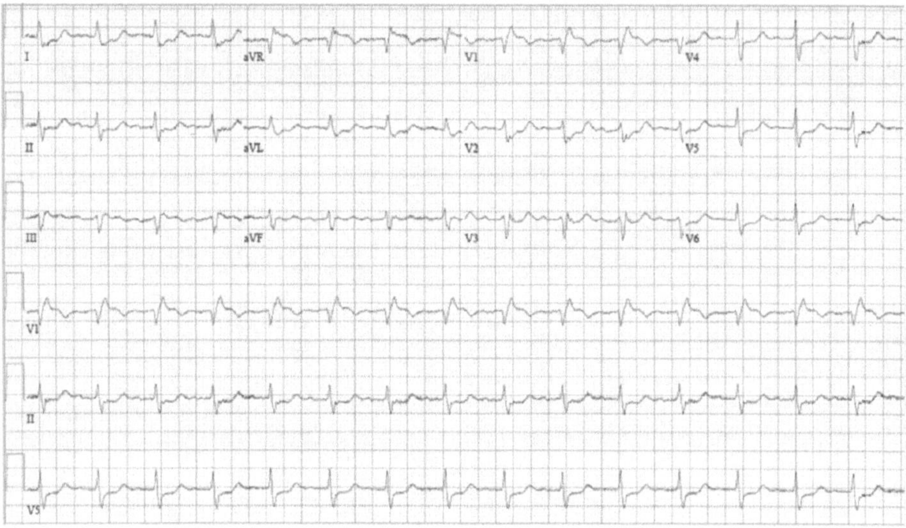

FIGURE 9.42

Rhythm: Sinus rhythm
Rate: 98 BPM
Axis: Normal (Physiologic)
Intervals: PR-interval >200 ms (1st Degree AV delay)
P-wave: Normal
QRS Complex: Right bundle branch block (RBBB)
T-wave: T-wave inversion (TWI) in Lead V1, ST-segment depressions (STDs) in Leads II, III, aVF, and V4–V6
Infarct: None

This ECG demonstrates sinus rhythm as the P-waves in Leads I, II, and aVF are positive. Also present is a right bundle branch block (RBBB) best appreciated in Leads V1 and V2, with a typical rsR'-wave in Lead V1, a slurred S-wave in Lead V6, and a total QRS complex duration of >120 ms. Additionally, there is at least a 50 ms delay in the onset of the intrinsicoid deflection (beginning of the QRS complex to the peak of the R-wave) in Leads V1 and V2. There is an associated T-wave inversion (TWI) in Lead V1, which is typically seen with RBBB. The PR interval is >200 ms, which is indicative of a 1st degree atrioventricular (AV) delay. There are ST-segment depressions (STDs) in Leads II, III, aVF, and V4–V6.

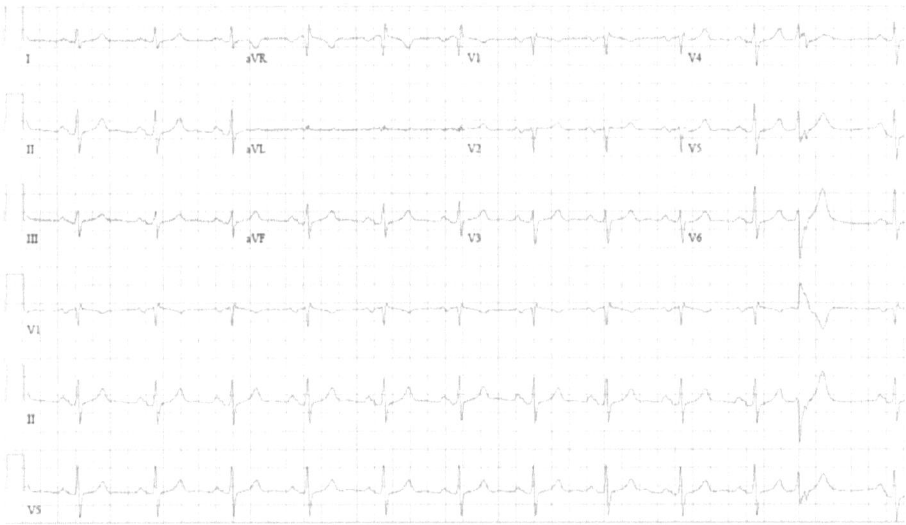

FIGURE 9.43

Rhythm: Sinus rhythm
Rate: 74 BPM
Axis: Normal (Physiologic)
Intervals: Borderline PR-interval >200 ms (1st Degree AV delay)
P-wave: Left atrial abnormality (LAA)
QRS Complex: Incomplete right bundle branch block (iRBBB)
T-wave: T-wave inversion (TWI) in Lead V1
Infarct: None

This ECG demonstrates sinus rhythm as the P-waves in Leads I, II, and aVF are positive, the P-wave in Lead V1 is biphasic. This tracing demonstrates an rSR' morphology in Leads V1 and V2, and is similar in morphology to a complete right bundle branch block (RBBB). However, the QRS complex duration is between 90 ms and 120 ms in duration, rather than the >120 ms that would be diagnostic for a complete RBBB. As such, this tracing is most consistent with an incomplete RBBB (iRBBB). There is a borderline 1st degree atrioventricular (AV) delay, as the PR-interval is ~200 ms in duration. The P-wave duration is borderline at ~120 ms, and the P-wave in Lead II demonstrates "notching (P-mitrale)," suggesting an LAA is present. The 11th beat on the rhythm strip corresponds to a premature ventricular contraction (PVC), followed by a compensatory pause.

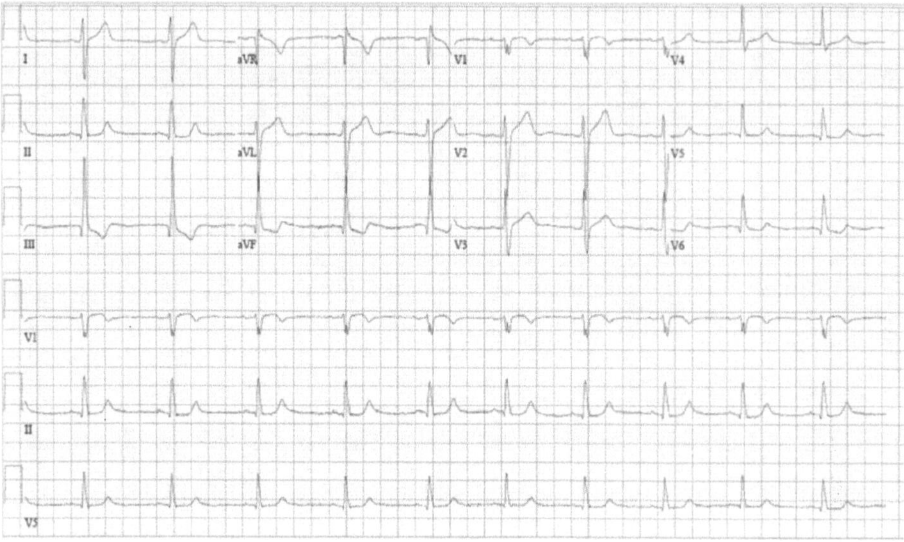

FIGURE 9.44

Rhythm: Sinus rhythm
Rate: 62 BPM
Axis: Right axis deviation (RAD)
Intervals: ST-segment depressions (STDs) in Leads II, III, aVF, V5, and V6
P-wave: Normal
QRS Complex: Left posterior hemiblock (LPH)
T-wave: T-wave inversions (TWIs) in Leads III and aVF
Infarct: None

This ECG demonstrates sinus rhythm as the P-waves in Leads I, II, and aVF are positive, the P-wave in Lead V1 is biphasic. A right axis deviation (RAD) is present, as the S-wave in Lead I is greater in amplitude than the corresponding R-wave, while the QRS complex in Leads II and aVF are positive in amplitude. Additionally, there is an rS-wave present in Leads I and aVL, a qR-wave in Lead III, and a QRS complex that is between 80 ms and 100 ms in duration. This pattern is demonstrative of a left posterior fascicular block (LPFB), which is also known as a left posterior hemiblock (LPH). Sinus arrhythmia is present as well, which is defined as the presence of sinus rhythm with a >120 ms variation in the RR interval. The relative inhibition of vagal tone during inspiration enables an increase in heart rate (HR), with the physiology being reversed during exhalation. Also noted are T-wave inversions (TWIs) along Leads III and aVF with associated ST-segment depressions (STDs), which may be concerning for ischemia.

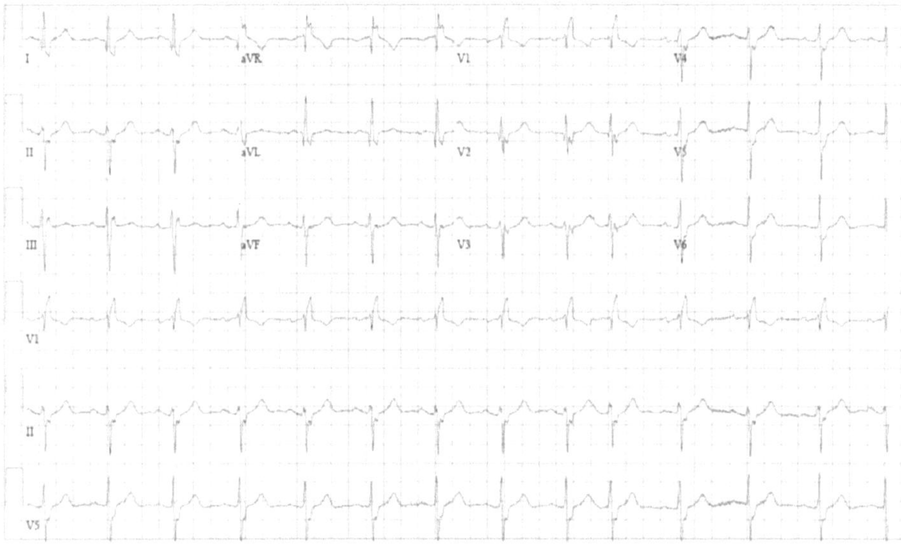

FIGURE 9.45

Rhythm: Sinus rhythm
Rate: 82 BPM
Axis: Left axis deviation (LAD)
Intervals: Borderline PR-interval >200 ms (1st Degree AV delay); QRS complex duration >120 ms
P-wave: Normal
QRS Complex: Right bundle branch block (RBBB); Left anterior hemiblock (LAH); Bifascicular block (BFB)
T-wave: T-wave inversion (TWI) in Lead V1
Infarct: None

This ECG demonstrates sinus rhythm as the P-waves in Leads I, II, and aVF are positive, the P-wave in Lead V1 is biphasic. A left axis deviation (LAD) is present, as the R-wave in Lead I is greater in amplitude than the corresponding S-wave, while the QRS complex in Leads II and aVF are negative in amplitude. Additionally, there is an rS-wave present in Leads I and aVL, a qR-wave in Lead III, and a QRS complex that is >120 ms in duration. This pattern is demonstrative of a left anterior fascicular block (LAFB), which is also known as a left anterior hemiblock (LAH). Also noted is an rSR' morphology in Leads V1 and V2, which is indicative of a complete right bundle branch block (RBBB). Collectively, the presence of an RBBB and an LAH in the same ECG is diagnostic for a bifascicular block (BFB). The T-wave inversion (TWI) in Lead V1 is a consequence of the RBBB. Finally, there is a borderline 1st degree atrioventricular (AV) delay, as the PR-interval is ~200 ms in duration. The 10th beat on the rhythm strip is consistent with a premature atrial contraction (PAC).

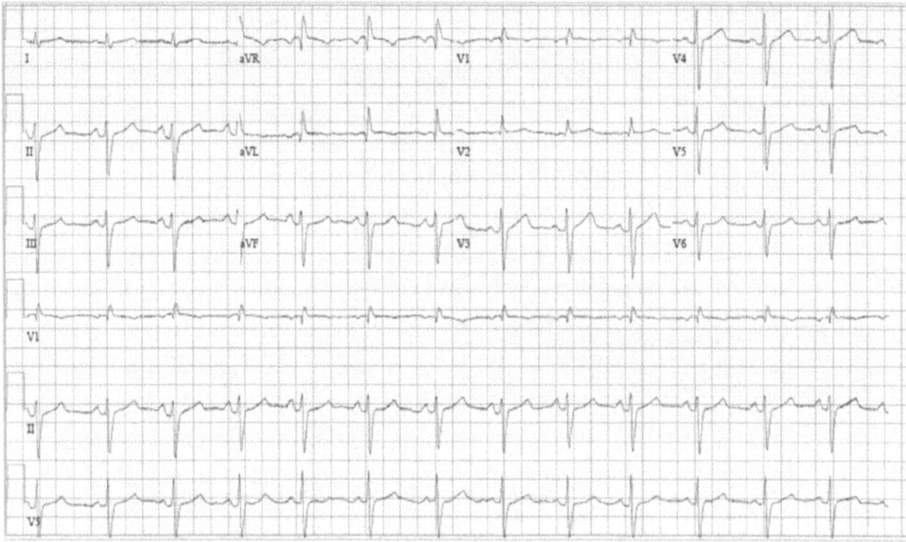

FIGURE 9.46

Rhythm: Sinus rhythm
Rate: 77 BPM
Axis: Left axis deviation (LAD)
Intervals: Normal
P-wave: Normal
QRS Complex: Incomplete RBBB (iRBBB); Left anterior hemiblock (LAH)
T-wave: T-wave inversion (TWI) in Lead V1
Infarct: None

This ECG demonstrates sinus rhythm as the P-waves in Leads I, II, and aVF are positive, the P-wave in Lead V1 is biphasic. A left axis deviation (LAD) is present, as the R-wave in Lead I is greater in amplitude than the corresponding S-wave, while the QRS complex in Leads II and aVF are negative in amplitude. Additionally, there is an rS-wave present in Leads I and aVL, a qR-wave in Lead III, and a QRS complex that is between 90 ms and 120 ms in duration. This pattern is demonstrative of a left anterior fascicular block (LAFB), which is also known as a left anterior hemiblock (LAH). Also noted is an rSR' morphology in Leads V1 and V2, which in the setting of a QRS complex duration between 90 ms and 120 ms is consistent with an incomplete right bundle branch block (iRBBB). The T-wave inversion (TWI) in Lead V1 is due to the iRBBB.

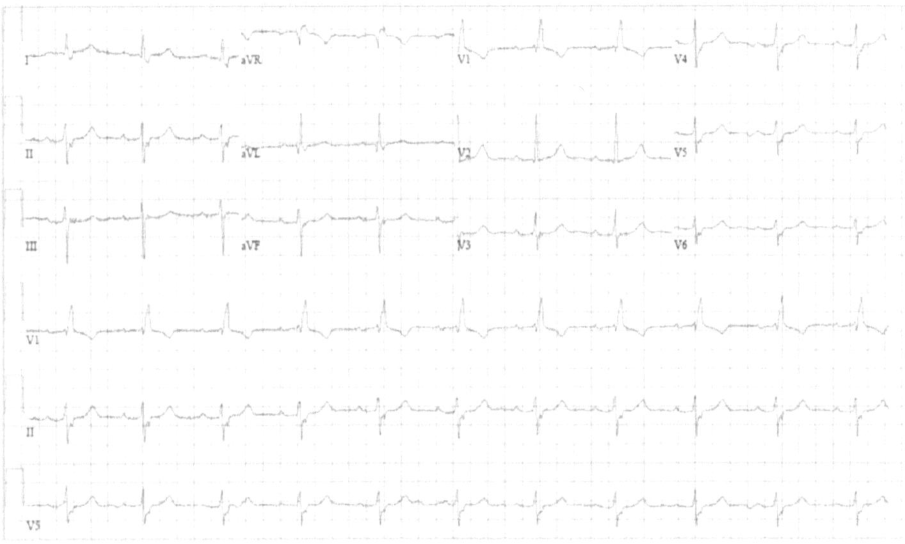

FIGURE 9.47

Rhythm: Sinus rhythm
Rate: 66 BPM
Axis: Left axis deviation (LAD)
Intervals: PR-interval >200 ms (1st Degree AV delay); QRS complex duration >120 ms
P-wave: Normal
QRS Complex: Complete RBBB (RBBB); Left anterior hemiblock (LAH); Bifascicular block (BFB)
T-wave: T-wave inversion (TWI) in Lead V1
Infarct: None

This ECG demonstrates sinus rhythm as the P-waves in Leads I, II, and aVF are positive, the P-wave in Lead V1 is biphasic. A left axis deviation (LAD) is present, as the R-wave in Lead I is greater in amplitude than the corresponding S-wave, while the QRS complex in Leads II and aVF are negative in amplitude. Additionally, there is an rS-wave present in Leads I and aVL, a qR-wave in Lead III, and a QRS complex that is >120 ms in duration. This pattern is demonstrative of a left anterior fascicular block (LAFB), which is also known as a left anterior hemiblock (LAH). Also noted is an rSR' morphology in Lead V1, which is indicative of a complete right bundle branch block (RBBB). Additionally, there is a 1st degree atrioventricular (AV) delay, as the PR-interval is >200 ms in duration. Collectively, the presence of an RBBB and an LAH in the same ECG is diagnostic for a bifascicular block (BFB). The T-wave inversion (TWI) in Lead V1 is a consequence of the RBBB.

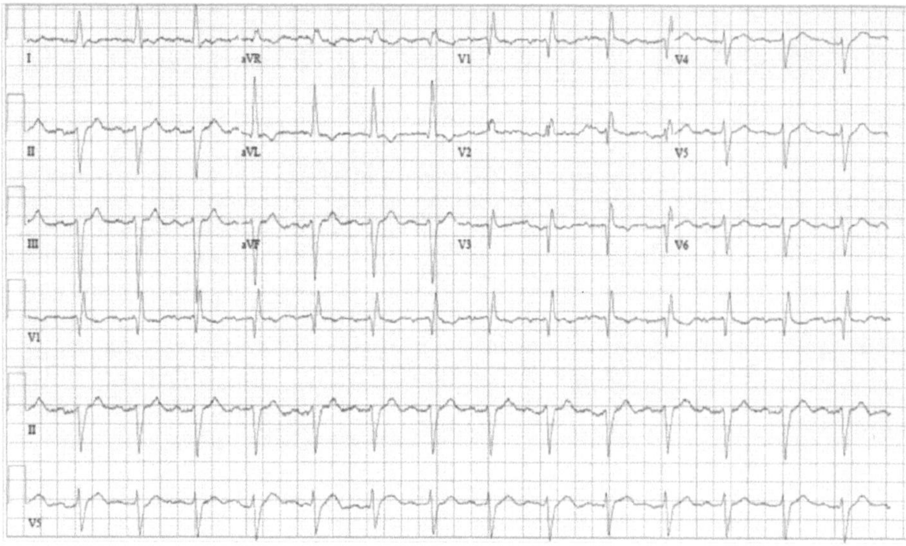

FIGURE 9.48

Rhythm: Sinus rhythm
Rate: 84 BPM
Axis: Left axis deviation (LAD)
Intervals: PR-interval >200 ms (1st Degree AV delay); QRS complex duration >120 ms
P-wave: Normal
QRS Complex: Right bundle branch block (RBBB); Left anterior hemiblock (LAH); Bifascicular block (BFB)
T-wave: T-wave inversions (TWIs) in Leads V1, I, and aVL
Infarct: None

This ECG demonstrates sinus rhythm as the P-waves in Leads I, II, and aVF are positive, the P-wave in Lead V1 is biphasic. A left axis deviation (LAD) is present, as the R-wave in Lead I is greater in amplitude than the corresponding S-wave, while the QRS complex in Leads II and aVF are negative in amplitude. Additionally, there is an rS-wave present in Leads I and aVL, a qR-wave in Lead III, and a QRS complex that is >120 ms in duration. This pattern is demonstrative of a left anterior fascicular block (LAFB), which is also known as a left anterior hemiblock (LAH). Also noted is an rSR' morphology in Leads V1 and V2, which is indicative of a complete right bundle branch block (RBBB). Additionally, there is a 1st degree atrioventricular (AV) delay, as the PR-interval is >200 ms in duration. Collectively, the presence of an RBBB and an LAH in the same ECG is diagnostic for a bifascicular block (BFB). Also present are T-wave inversions (TWIs) in Leads I and aVL, concerning for ischemia. The TWI in Lead V1 is a consequence of the RBBB.

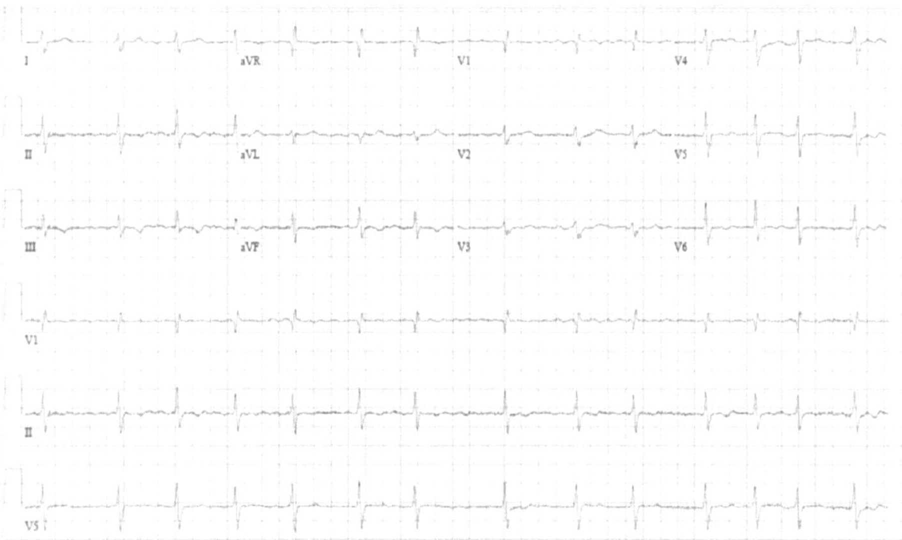

FIGURE 9.49

Rhythm: Atrial fibrillation with a controlled ventricular response (CVR)
Rate: 84 BPM
Axis: Right axis deviation (RAD)
Intervals: Normal
P-wave: Not applicable
QRS Complex: Poor R-wave progression (PRWP)
T-waves: T-wave inversions (TWIs) in Leads II, III, and aVF
Infarct: None

This ECG demonstrates a lack of discernable P-waves amidst a random oscillation of electrical activity along the baseline, which is consistent with atrial fibrillation (Afib). The f-waves (fibrillatory waves) are characterized by random deflections that vary in terms of duration, amplitude, and morphology. This is associated with an irregularly irregular RR interval with a controlled ventricular response (CVR) due to the ventricular heart rate (HR) between 60 BPM and 100 BPM. Also noted are T-wave inversions (TWIs) along Leads II, III, and aVF, concerning for ischemia. There is an associated poor R-wave progression (PRWP) along the precordial leads, as the QRS complex does not become positive until Lead V6, with the isoelectric point between Leads V5 and V6. A right axis deviation (RAD) is noted, as the S-wave in Lead I is greater in amplitude than the corresponding R-wave, while the QRS complex in Leads II and aVF are positive in amplitude.

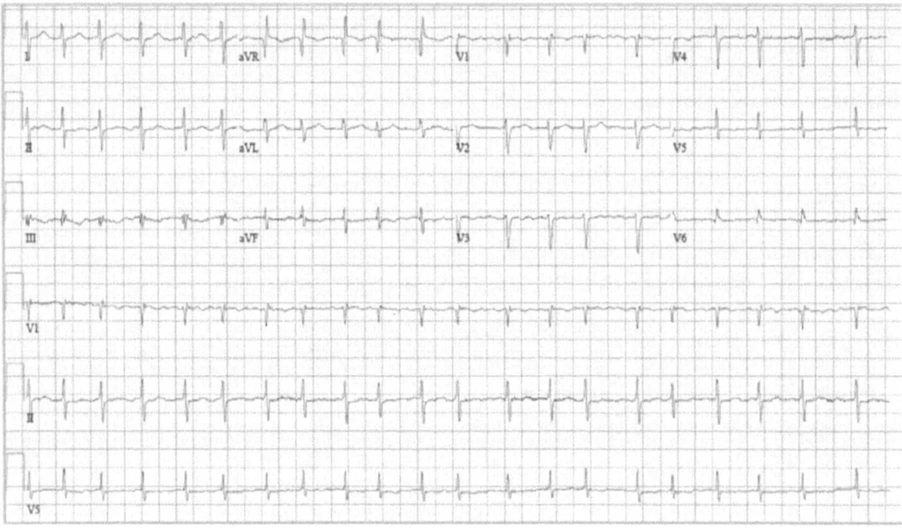

FIGURE 9.50

Rhythm: Atrial fibrillation with a rapid ventricular response (RVR)
Rate: 126 BPM
Axis: Extreme right axis deviation (RAD)
Intervals: Normal
P-waves: Not applicable
QRS Complex: RV Conduction delay; Poor R-wave progression (PRWP)
T-waves: T-wave inversions (TWIs) in Leads III and aVF
Infarct: None

This ECG demonstrates a lack of discernable P-waves amidst a random oscillation of electrical activity along the baseline, which is consistent with atrial fibrillation (Afib). The f-waves (fibrillatory waves) are characterized by random deflections that vary in terms of duration, amplitude, and morphology. This is associated with an irregularly irregular RR interval with a rapid ventricular response (RVR), due to the ventricular heart rate >100 BPM. The QRS axis on this tracing is a Northwestern axis (also known as an extreme right axis deviation or a superior axis) due to the S-waves in Leads I, II, and aVF being > in amplitude than their corresponding R-waves. There is a right ventricular (RV) conduction delay present, as the QRS complex adopts a right bundle branch block (RBBB) morphology, but is <100 ms in duration. Additionally, there are T-wave inversions (TWIs) along Leads III and aVF, concerning for ischemia. There is an associated poor R-wave progression (PRWP) along the precordial leads, as the QRS complex does not become positive until Lead V5, with the isoelectric point between Leads V4 and V5.

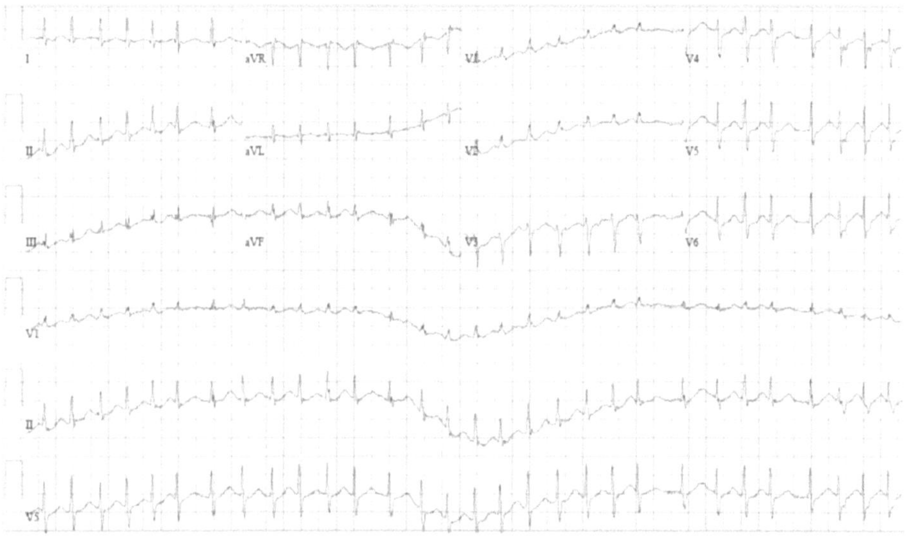

FIGURE 9.51

Rhythm: Atrial fibrillation with a rapid ventricular response (RVR)
Rate: 180 BPM
Axis: Normal (Physiologic)
Intervals: Normal
P-waves: Not applicable
QRS Complex: Normal
T-waves: Normal
Infarct: None

This ECG demonstrates a lack of discernable P-waves amidst a random oscillation of electrical activity along the baseline, which is consistent with atrial fibrillation (Afib). The f-waves (fibrillatory waves) are characterized by random deflections that vary in terms of duration, amplitude, and morphology. This is associated with an irregularly irregular RR interval with a rapid ventricular response (RVR), due to the ventricular heart rate >100 BPM. Afib with particularly rapid ventricular conduction (>180 BPM in this tracing) may cause the RR interval to "regularize," causing the differences in adjacent RR intervals to be minimized. Incidentally noted is extensive motion artifact, manifesting as a wandering baseline, that is most apparent when viewed along the rhythm strips. The wavy nature of the baseline is due to patient movement.

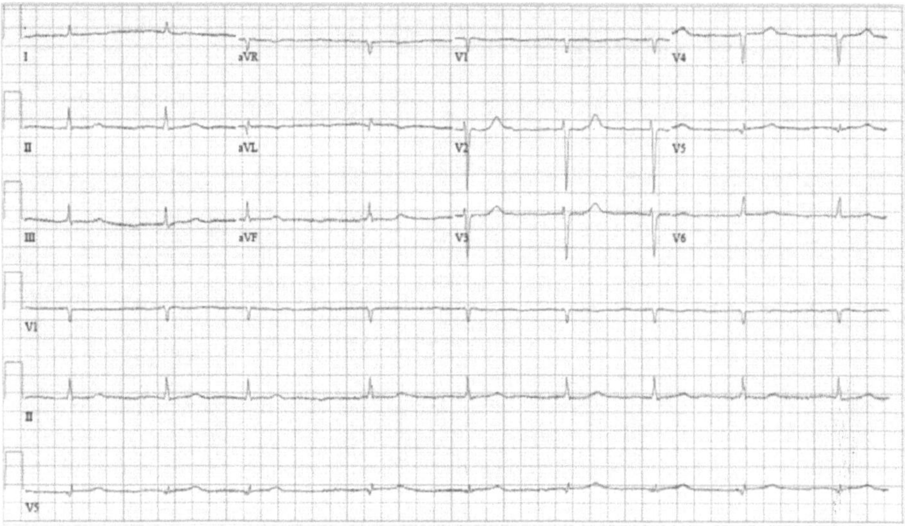

FIGURE 9.52

Rhythm: Atrial fibrillation with a slow ventricular response (SVR)
Rate: 54 BPM
Axis: Normal (Physiologic)
Intervals: Normal
P-waves: Not applicable
QRS Complex: Poor R-wave progression (PRWP)
T-waves: Normal
Infarct: None

This ECG demonstrates a lack of discernable P-waves amidst a random oscillation of electrical activity along the baseline, which is consistent with atrial fibrillation (Afib). The f-waves (fibrillatory waves) are characterized by random deflections that vary in terms of duration, amplitude, and morphology. This is associated with an irregularly irregular RR interval with a slow ventricular response (SVR), due to the ventricular heart rate <60 BPM. There is an associated poor R-wave progression (PRWP) along the precordial leads, as the QRS complex does not become positive until Lead V6, with the isoelectric point between Leads V5 and V6.

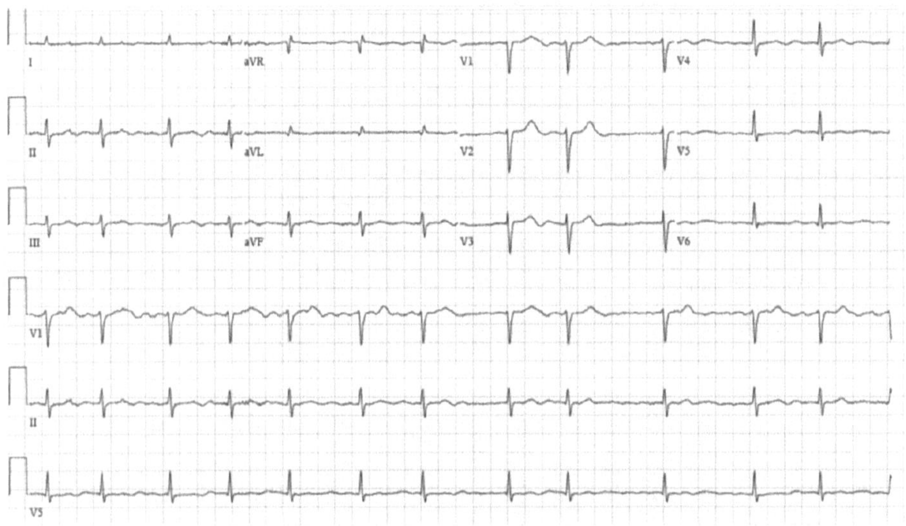

FIGURE 9.53

Rhythm: Atrial fibrillation with a controlled ventricular response (CVR)
Rate: 78 BPM
Axis: Normal (Physiologic)
Intervals: Normal
P-wave: Not applicable
QRS Complex: Normal
T-wave: Nonspecific T-wave abnormality in Leads I, III, aVF, aVL, V5, and V6
Infarct: None

This ECG demonstrates f-waves rather than P-waves, which is indicative of atrial fibrillation (Afib). The atrial rate being >300 beats per minute (BPM) and the different morphologies of the f-waves within any given lead also denote atrial fibrillation (Afib). With a ventricular rate between 60 BPM and 100 BPM, as is the case with this tracing, the proper terminology would be Afib with a controlled ventricular response (CVR). There is a nonspecific T-wave abnormality present along Leads I, III, aVF, aVL, V5, and V6.

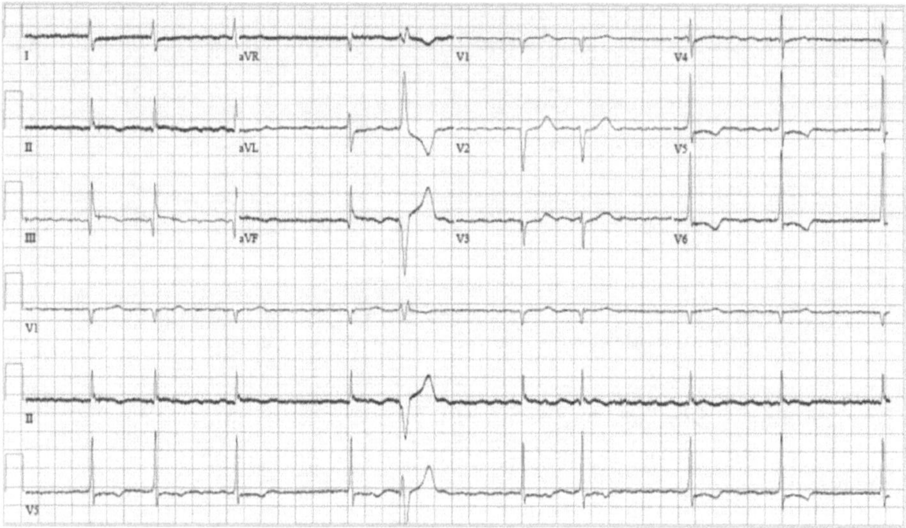

FIGURE 9.54

Rhythm: Coarse atrial fibrillation with a controlled ventricular response (CVR)
Rate: 60 BPM
Axis: Normal (Physiologic)
Intervals: <1 mm ST-segment elevations (STEs) in Leads II, III, and aVF
P-waves: Not applicable
QRS Complex: Pathological Q-waves in Leads V1–V3
T-waves: ST-segment depressions (STDs) and T-wave inversions (TWIs) in Leads V5 and V6
Infarct: Anteroseptal ST-segment elevation myocardial infarction (STEMI)

This ECG demonstrates a lack of discernable P-waves amidst a random oscillation of electrical activity along the baseline, which is consistent with atrial fibrillation (Afib). The f-waves (fibrillatory waves) are characterized by random deflections that vary in terms of duration, amplitude, and morphology. This is associated with an irregularly irregular RR interval with a controlled ventricular response (CVR), due to the ventricular heart rate between 60 BPM and 100 BPM. Specifically, there are periods of atrial activity that resemble the "sawtooth" pattern characteristic of "F-waves" (flutter waves) that are interspersed with a more chaotic baseline. This is consistent with "coarse" Afib, which is manifested by different fibrillatory wave (f-wave) morphologies within the same Lead. Also noted are <1 mm ST-segment elevations (STEs) in Leads II, III, and aVF with reciprocal ST-segment depressions (STDs) and T-wave inversions (TWIs) in Leads V5 and V6, demonstrative of an inferior wall ST-segment myocardial infarction (STEMI). The 5th beat on the rhythm strip is a premature ventricular complex (PVC).

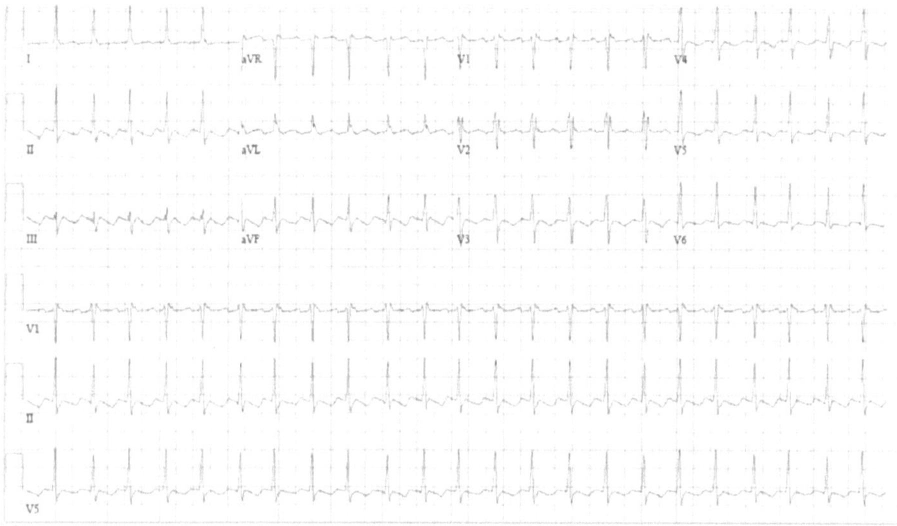

FIGURE 9.55

Rhythm: 2:1 Atrial flutter with a rapid ventricular response (RVR)
Rate: 138 BPM
Axis: Normal (Physiological)
Intervals: Normal
P-wave: Not-applicable
QRS Complex: Incomplete right bundle branch block (iRBBB)
T-wave: Not applicable
Infarct: None

This ECG demonstrates a lack of discernable P-waves and is instead marked by "saw-tooth" deflections throughout the baseline of the tracing, indicative of atrial flutter. These F-waves (flutter waves) are characterized by the aforementioned "sawtooth" or "picket fence" morphology that have the same duration, amplitude, and morphology within the same Lead. Moreover, the lack of a clear isoelectric segment within the RR interval is also indicative of atrial flutter. There are two F-waves for every QRS complex, resulting in a fixed 2:1 atrioventricular conduction ratio and, as a result, a regular RR interval. This tracing displays a rapid ventricular response (RVR), due to the ventricular heart rate >100 BPM. Also noted is an rSR' morphology in Leads V1 and V2, which in the setting of a QRS complex duration between 90 ms and 120 ms is consistent with an incomplete right bundle branch block (iRBBB).

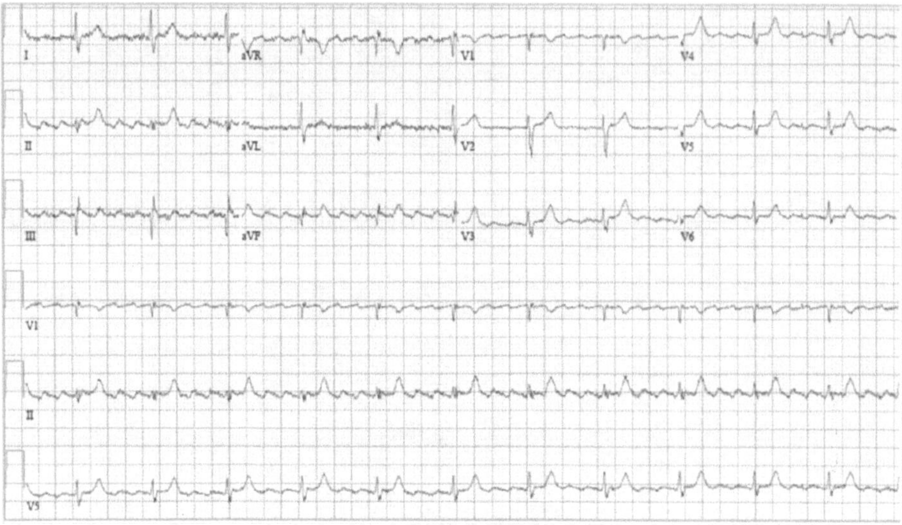

FIGURE 9.56

Rhythm: 4:1 Atrial flutter with a controlled ventricular response (CVR)
Rate: 66 BPM
Axis: Left axis deviation (LAD)
Intervals: Normal
P-wave: Not applicable
QRS Complex: Normal
T-wave: Not applicable
Infarct: Possible pathological Q-waves in Leads II, III, and aVF

This ECG demonstrates a lack of discernable P-waves and is instead marked by "saw-tooth" deflections throughout the baseline of the tracing, indicative of atrial flutter. These F-waves (flutter waves) are characterized by the aforementioned "sawtooth" or "picket fence" morphology that have the same duration, amplitude, and morphology within the same Lead. There are four F-waves for every QRS complex, resulting in a fixed 4:1 atrioventricular conduction ratio and, as a result, a regular RR interval. This tracing displays a controlled ventricular response (CVR), due to the ventricular heart rate between 60 BPM and 100 BPM. A left axis deviation (LAD) is present, as the R-wave in Lead I is greater in amplitude than the corresponding S-wave, while the QRS complex in Leads II and aVF are negative in amplitude. There may be pathological Q-waves in Leads II, III, and aVF.

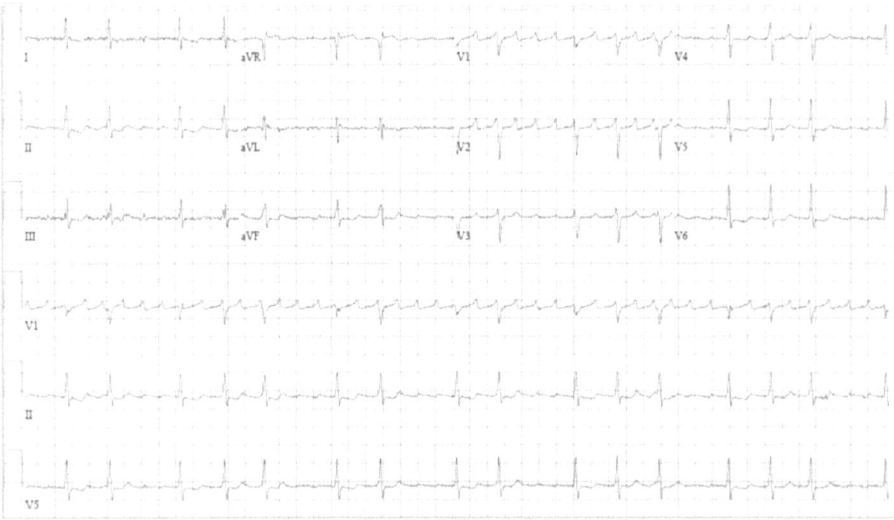

FIGURE 9.57

Rhythm: Atrial flutter with a controlled ventricular response (CVR) and a variable block
Rate: 96 BPM
Axis: Normal (Physiologic)
Intervals: Normal
P-wave: Not applicable
QRS Complex: Normal
T-wave: Not applicable
Infarct: None

This ECG demonstrates a lack of discernable P-waves and is instead marked by "sawtooth" deflections throughout the baseline of the tracing, indicative of atrial flutter. These F-waves (flutter waves) are characterized by the aforementioned "sawtooth" or "picket fence" morphology that have the same duration, amplitude, and morphology within the same Lead. There is a variable number of F-waves that occur prior to the next conducted QRS complex, resulting in a variable atrioventricular conduction ratio and, as a result, an irregular RR interval. This tracing displays a controlled ventricular response (CVR), due to the ventricular heart rate between 60 BPM and 100 BPM.

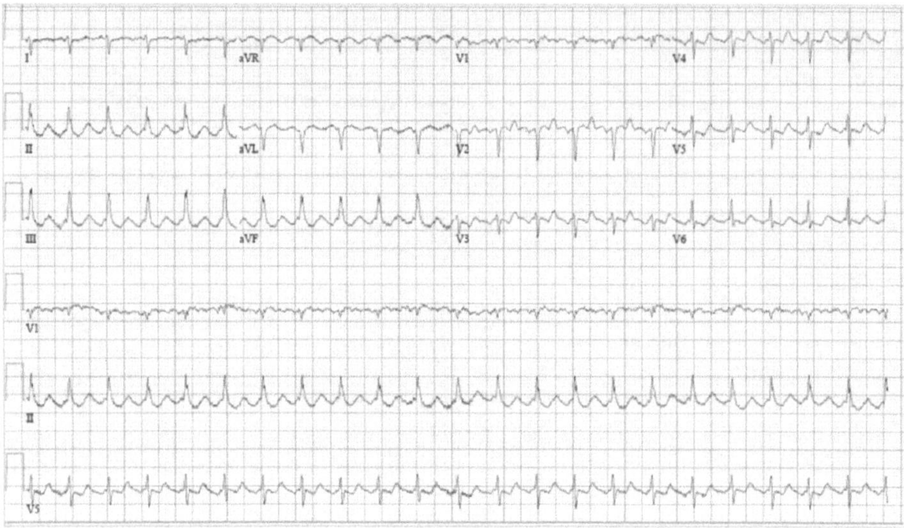

FIGURE 9.58

Rhythm: 2:1 Atrial flutter with a rapid ventricular response (RVR)
Rate: 138 BPM
Axis: Right axis deviation (RAD)
Intervals: Normal
P-wave: Not applicable
QRS Complex: Normal
T-wave: Not applicable
Infarct: None

This ECG demonstrates a lack of discernable P-waves and is instead marked by "sinusoidal" deflections throughout the baseline of the tracing, indicative of atrial flutter. These F-waves (flutter waves) are characterized by the aforementioned "sinusoidal" morphology that has the same duration, amplitude, and morphology within the same Lead. Furthermore, there is a lack of an isoelectric baseline between adjacent QRS complexes, which is expected for atrial flutter. There are two F-waves for every QRS complex, resulting in a fixed 2:1 atrioventricular conduction ratio and, as a result, a regular RR interval. This tracing displays a rapid ventricular response (RVR) due to the ventricular heart rate >100 BPM. A right axis deviation (RAD) is present, as the S-wave in Lead I is greater in amplitude than the corresponding R-wave, while the QRS complex in Leads II and aVF are positive in amplitude.

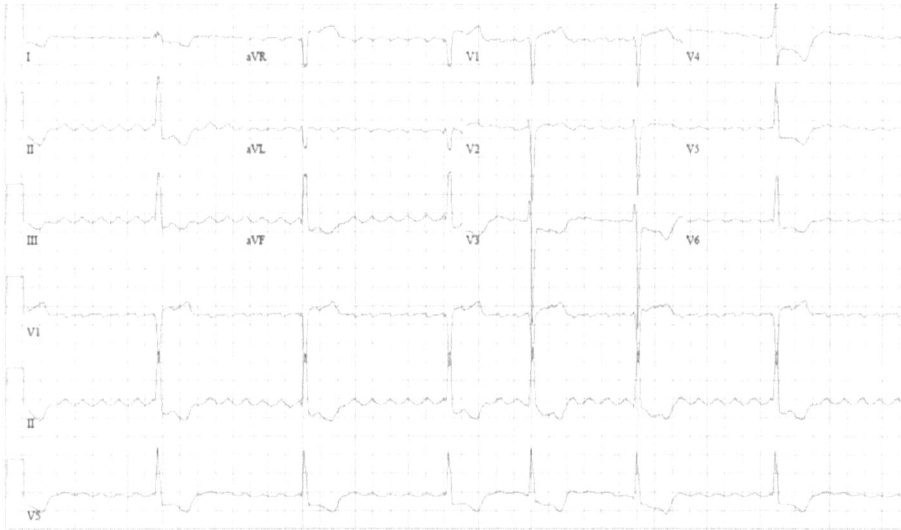

FIGURE 9.59

Rhythm: Atrial flutter with a slow ventricular response (SVR) with a variable block
Rate: 39 BPM
Axis: Normal (Physiologic)
Intervals: ST-segment depressions (STDs) in Leads II, III, aVF, V3–V6
P-wave: Not applicable
QRS Complex: Normal
T-wave: T-wave inversions (TWIs) along Leads II, III, aVF, and V3–V6
Infarct: None

This ECG demonstrates a lack of discernable P-waves and is instead marked by "sawtooth" deflections throughout the baseline of the tracing, indicative of atrial flutter. These F-waves (flutter waves) are characterized by the aforementioned "sawtooth" or "picket fence" morphology that have the same duration, amplitude, and morphology within the same Lead. There is a variable number of F-waves that occur prior to the next conducted QRS complex, resulting in a variable atrioventricular conduction ratio and, as a result, an irregular RR interval. There are ST-segment depressions (STDs) and T-wave inversions (TWIs) along Leads II, III, aVF, and V3–V6, which may be a repolarization abnormality associated with ventricular escape beats. This tracing displays a slow ventricular response (SVR) due to the ventricular heart rate 60 BPM.

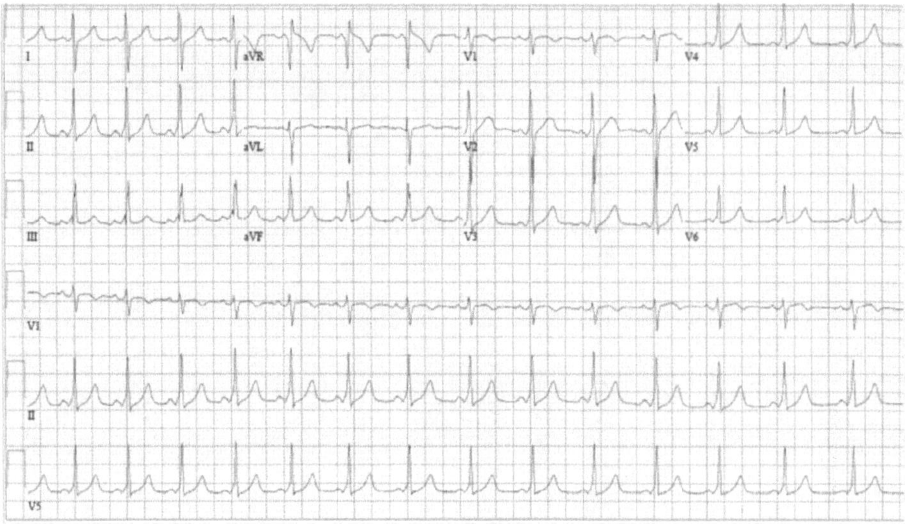

FIGURE 9.60

Rhythm: Sinus rhythm
Rate: 85 BPM
Axis: Right axis deviation (RAD)
Intervals: PR interval <120 ms, Delta wave
P-wave: Normal
QRS Complex: Narrow with slurred intrinsicoid deflection
T-wave: Normal
Infarct: None

This ECG demonstrates sinus rhythm, as the P-waves in Leads I, II, and aVF are positive, and the P-wave in Lead V1 is biphasic. The PR interval is short (<120 ms), and the QRS complex has a slurred intrinsicoid deflection; this is consistent with ventricular pre-excitation, specifically the Wolff–Parkinson–White pattern. Also present is a right axis deviation (RAD), as the S-wave in Lead I is greater in amplitude than the corresponding R-wave, while the QRS complex in Leads II and aVF are positive in amplitude. In the setting of pre-excitation, it is not feasible to comment on infarct pattern.

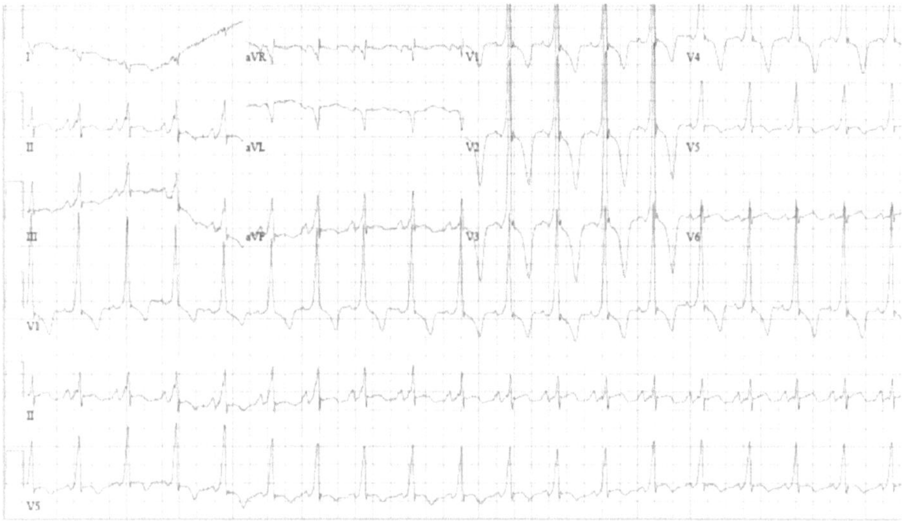

FIGURE 9.61

Rhythm: Sinus tachycardia
Rate: 114 BPM
Axis: Right axis deviation (RAD)
Intervals: PR interval <120 ms, Delta wave
P-wave: Normal
QRS Complex: Wide with slurred intrinsicoid deflection
T-wave: T-wave inversions (TWIs) along Leads V1–V5
Infarct: None

This ECG demonstrates sinus rhythm, as the P-waves in Leads I, II, and aVF are positive, and the P-wave in Lead V1 is biphasic. The PR interval is short (<120 ms), and the QRS complex has a slurred intrinsicoid deflection; this is consistent with ventricular pre-excitation, specifically the Wolff–Parkinson–White pattern. Furthermore, a right axis deviation (RAD) is present, as the S-wave in Lead I is greater in amplitude than the corresponding R-wave, while the QRS complex in Lead II is positive in polarity. There are T-wave inversions (TWIs) in Leads V1–V5, due to pre-excitation.

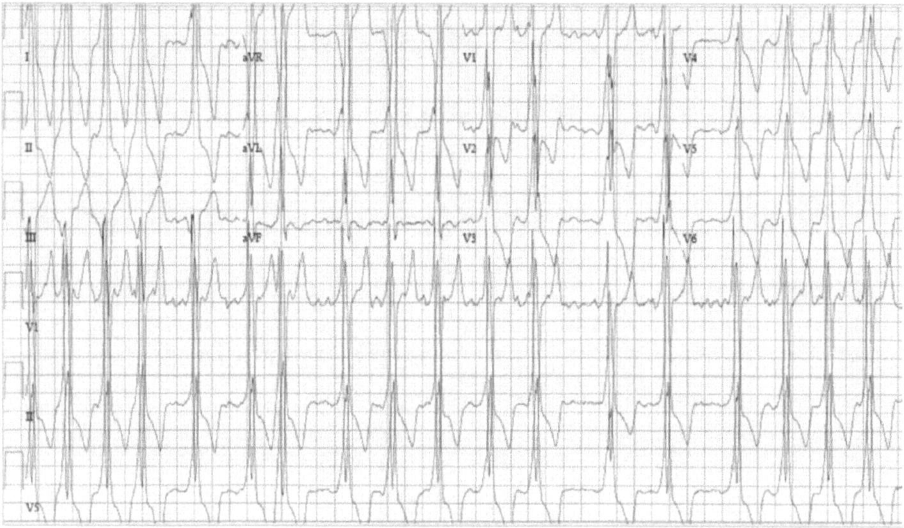

FIGURE 9.62

Rhythm: Pre-excited atrial fibrillation with a rapid ventricular response (RVR)
Rate: 112 BPM
Axis: Normal (Physiologic)
Intervals: Delta wave
P-wave: Not applicable
QRS Complex: Wide with slurred intrinsicoid deflection
T-wave: T-wave inversions (TWIs) along Leads V2–V6
Infarct: None

This ECG demonstrates a lack of discernable P-waves amidst a random oscillation of electrical activity along the baseline, which is consistent with atrial fibrillation (Afib). The f-waves (fibrillatory waves) are characterized by random deflections that vary in terms of duration, amplitude, and morphology. This is associated with an irregularly irregular RR interval with a rapid ventricular response (RVR), due to the ventricular heart rate >100 BPM. The wide QRS duration (>120 ms), slurred intrinsicoid deflection, and subtle variation in QRS widths imply underlying pre-excitation, such as from the Wolff–Parkinson–White pattern. There are T-wave inversions (TWIs) in Leads V2–V6, due to pre-excitation.

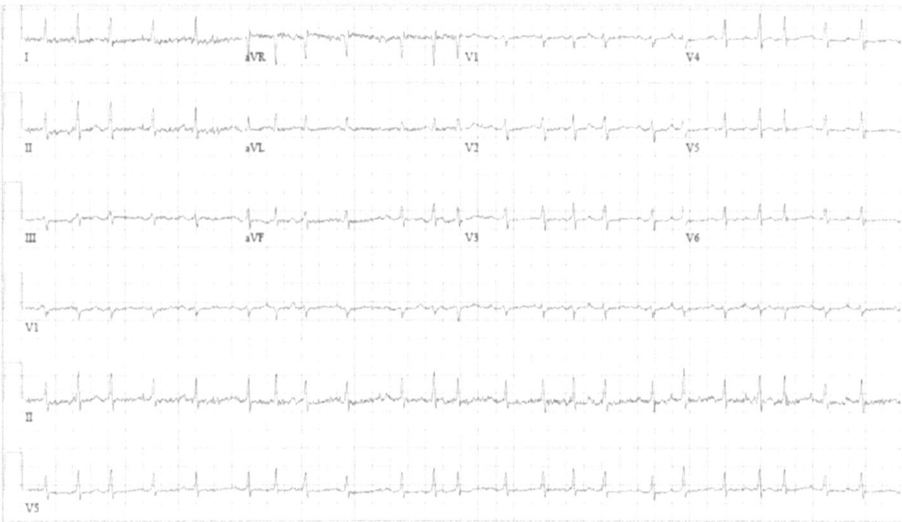

FIGURE 9.63

Rhythm: Multifocal atrial tachycardia (MAT)
Rate: 138 BPM
Axis: Normal (Physiologic)
Intervals: Normal
P-wave: >3 morphologies within the same Lead
QRS Complex: Low voltage in the precordial Leads
T-wave: Nonspecific T-wave flattening in Leads I, II, III, aVL, aVF, and V4–V6
Infarct: None

This ECG demonstrates an irregular rhythm with a tachycardic rate with at least three P-wave morphologies in the same Lead, meeting criteria for multifocal atrial tachycardia (MAT). There is nonspecific T-wave flattening in Leads I, II, III, aVL, aVF, and V4–V6. Additionally, the amplitude of the QRS complex in the precordial Leads does not exceed two large boxes (10 mm), which is consistent with low voltage.

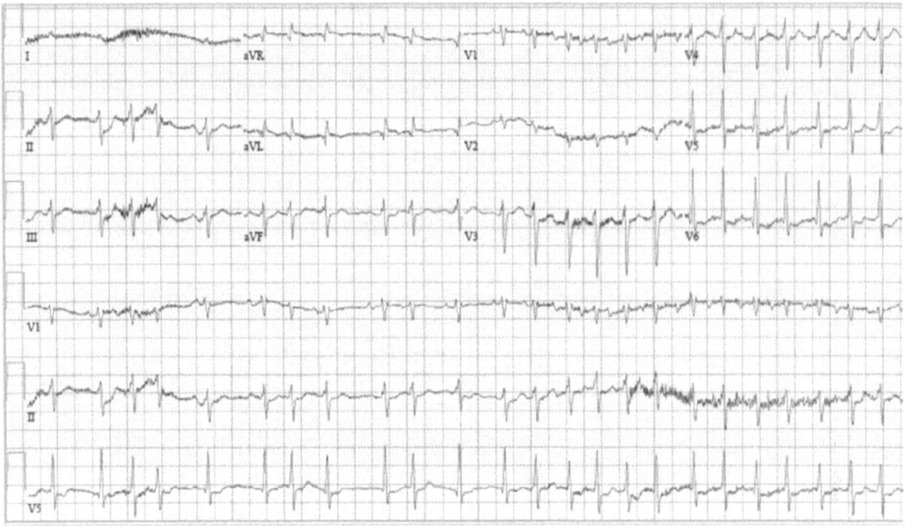

FIGURE 9.64

Rhythm: Multifocal atrial tachycardia (MAT), paroxysmal atrial tachycardia (pAT)
Rate: 130 BPM
Axis: Left axis deviation (LAD)
Intervals: Normal
P-wave: >3 morphologies within the same Lead
QRS Complex: Poor R-wave progression (PRWP)
T-wave: Nonspecific T-wave flattening in Leads I, II, III, aVL, aVF, and V4–V6
Infarct: None

This ECG demonstrates an irregular rhythm with a tachycardic rate with at least three P-wave morphologies in the same Lead, meeting criteria for multifocal atrial tachycardia (MAT). Additionally, the rhythm organizes after the 11th beat into an atrial tachyarrhythmia with one P-wave morphology known as paroxysmal atrial tachycardia (pAT). There is a left axis deviation (LAD) present in this ECG as well, as indicated by the R-wave amplitude > S-wave amplitude in Lead I, in contrast to the R-wave amplitude < S-wave amplitude in Lead II. There is a nonspecific T-wave flattening in Leads I, II, III, aVL, aVF, and V4–V6. There is an associated poor R-wave progression (PRWP) along the precordial leads, as the QRS complex does not become positive until Lead V5, with the isoelectric point between Leads V4 and V5.

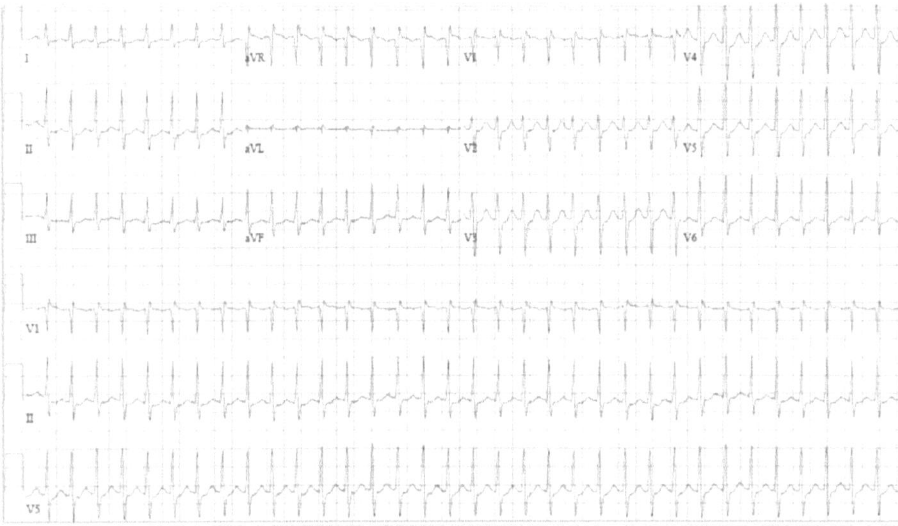

FIGURE 9.65

Rhythm: Supraventricular tachycardia (SVT) [Short-RP tachycardia]
Rate: 204 BPM
Axis: Normal (Physiologic)
Intervals: Normal
P-wave: Retrograde, inverted
QRS Complex: Normal
T-wave: Diffuse upsloping ST-segment depressions
Infarct: None

This ECG demonstrates a narrow-complex tachycardia with a ventricular heart rate (HR) in excess of 200 BPM. There are no antecedent P-waves prior to the QRS complex, but there are inverted P-waves present after the QRS complex. This rhythm would be classified as supraventricular tachycardia (SVT), and more precisely, a short-RP tachycardia. The amount of time between the R-wave and the inverted P-wave is shorter than that from the inverted P-wave to the next R-wave, hence the name. A pseudo R'-wave may be seen in Lead V1, which gives the appearance of an incomplete right bundle branch block (iRBBB). There are diffuse, upsloping ST-segment depressions, which are more consistent with decreased coronary perfusion from the rapid HR, rather than ischemia.

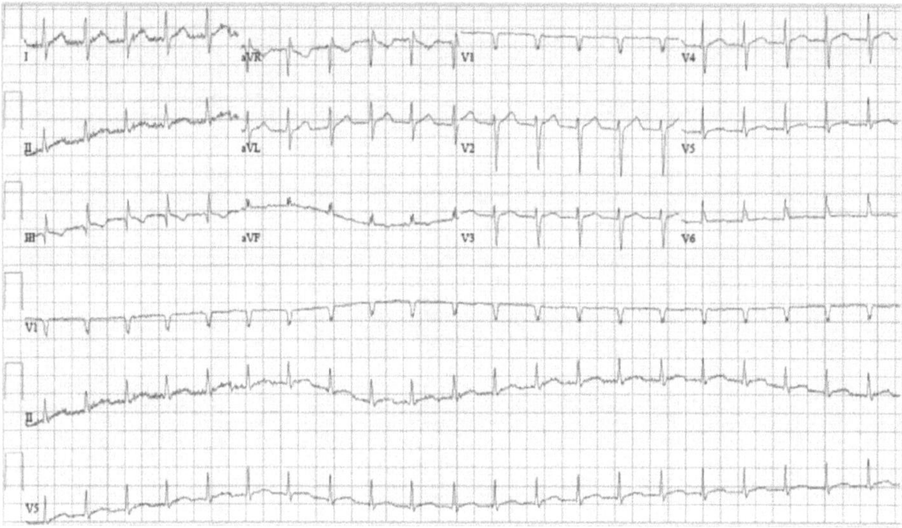

FIGURE 9.66

Rhythm: Supraventricular tachycardia (SVT) [Short-RP tachycardia]
Rate: 127 BPM
Axis: Normal (Physiologic)
Intervals: Normal
P-wave: Retrograde, inverted
QRS Complex: Normal
T-wave: T-wave inversion (TWI) in Leads III and aVF
Infarct: None

This ECG demonstrates a narrow-complex tachycardia with a ventricular heart rate (HR) of more than 120 BPM. There are no antecedent P-waves prior to the QRS complex, but there are inverted P-waves present after the QRS complex. This rhythm would be classified as supraventricular tachycardia (SVT), and more precisely, a short-RP tachycardia. The amount of time between the R-wave and the inverted P-wave is shorter than that from the inverted P-wave to the next R-wave, hence the name. A pseudo R'-wave is seen in Leads V1–V3, which may give off the appearance of an incomplete right bundle branch block (iRBBB). There are T-wave inversions (TWIs) in Leads III and aVF, which may be consistent with ischemia.

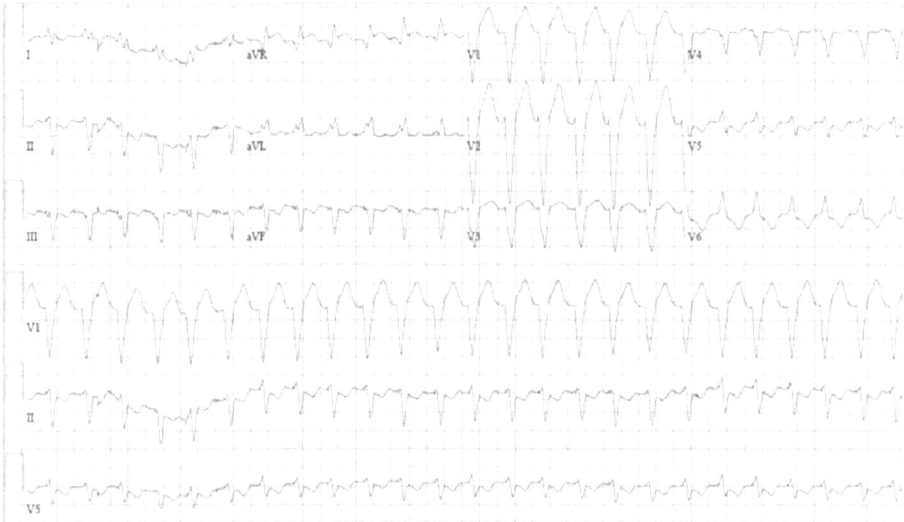

FIGURE 9.67

Rhythm: Supraventricular tachycardia (SVT) [Short-RP tachycardia] with left bundle branch block (LBBB) aberrancy
Rate: 150 BPM
Axis: Left axis deviation (LAD)
Intervals: Normal
P-wave: Not Applicable
QRS Complex: Left bundle branch block (LBBB)
T-wave: T-wave inversions (TWIs) in Leads II, III, aVF, and V4–V6
Infarct: Pathological Q-waves in Leads III and aVF

This ECG demonstrates a wide-complex tachycardia with a left bundle branch block (LBBB) morphology. By Brugada criteria, the patient does have RS-waves, and the R-S nadir is <80 ms. Moreover, there is no evidence of atrioventricular (AV) dissociation, and the LBBB has typical morphologies in both Leads V1 and V6. As such, this rhythm is consistent with supraventricular tachycardia (SVT) with LBBB aberrancy. This SVT is considered a short RP-tachycardia, as the P-wave is not visible. There is a left axis deviation (LAD) present in this ECG as well, as indicated by the R-wave amplitude > S-wave amplitude in Lead I, in contrast to the R-wave amplitude < S-wave amplitude in Lead II. There are pathological Q-waves along Leads III and aVF, consistent with a previous myocardial infarction (MI). There are T-wave inversions (TWIs) in Leads II, III, aVF, and V4–V6.

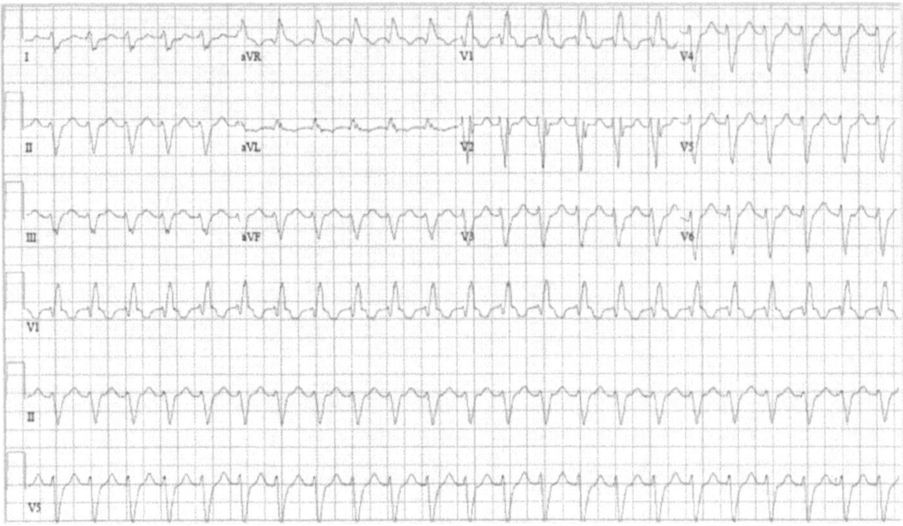

FIGURE 9.68

Rhythm: Supraventricular tachycardia (SVT) [Short-RP tachycardia] with right bundle branch block (RBBB) aberrancy
Rate: 138 BPM
Axis: Northwestern axis deviation
Intervals: Normal
P-wave: Not applicable
QRS Complex: Right bundle branch block (RBBB)
T-wave: T-wave inversion (TWI) in Lead aVL
Infarct: None

This ECG demonstrates a wide-complex tachycardia with a right bundle branch block (RBBB) morphology. By Brugada criteria, the patient does have RS-waves, and the R-S nadir is <80 ms. Moreover, there is no evidence of atrioventricular (AV) dissociation, and the RBBB has a typical morphology in Lead V1. Although the RBBB morphology in Lead V6 is atypical, morphological criteria for VT are not met, and as such, this tracing represents a supraventricular tachycardia (SVT) with RBBB aberrancy. The QRS axis on this tracing is a Northwestern axis (also known as an extreme right axis, or a superior axis), due to the S-waves in both Leads I and II being greater in amplitude than their respective R-waves. There is a T-wave inversion (TWI) of Lead aVL, without any pathological Q-waves.

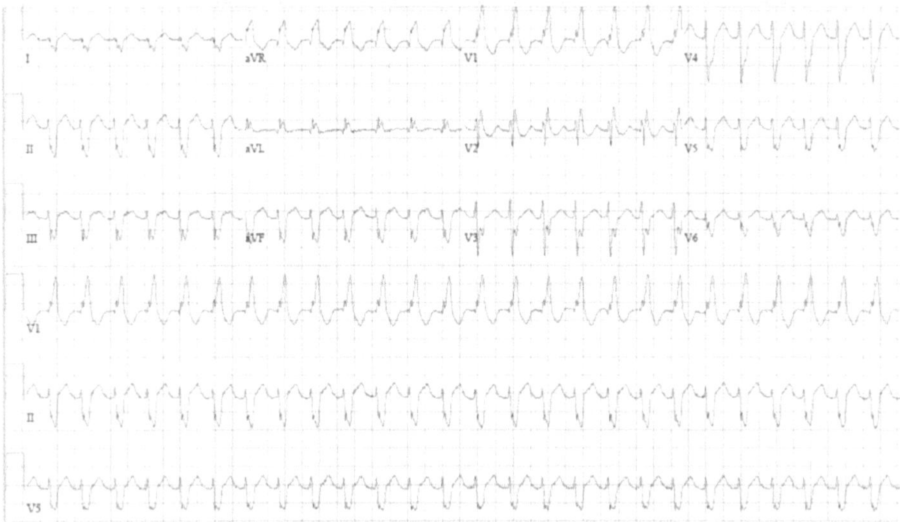

FIGURE 9.69

Rhythm: Supraventricular tachycardia (SVT) [Short-RP tachycardia] with right bundle branch block (RBBB) aberrancy
Rate: 156 BPM
Axis: Northwestern axis deviation
Intervals: Normal
P-wave: Not applicable
QRS Complex: Right bundle branch block (RBBB)
T-wave: None
Infarct: None

This ECG demonstrates a wide-complex tachycardia with a right bundle branch block (RBBB) morphology. By Brugada criteria, the patient does have RS-waves, and the R-S nadir is <80 ms. Moreover, there is no evidence of atrioventricular (AV) dissociation, and the RBBB has a typical morphology in Lead V1. The rSR' in Lead V1 is typical, as the r-wave is smaller in amplitude than the R'-wave. Although the RBBB morphology in Lead V6 is atypical (S-wave amplitude > R-wave amplitude), morphological criteria for VT are not met, and as such, this tracing represents a supraventricular tachycardia (SVT) with RBBB aberrancy. The QRS axis on this tracing is a Northwestern axis (also known as an extreme right axis, or a superior axis), due to the S-waves in both Leads I and II being greater in amplitude than their respective R-waves.

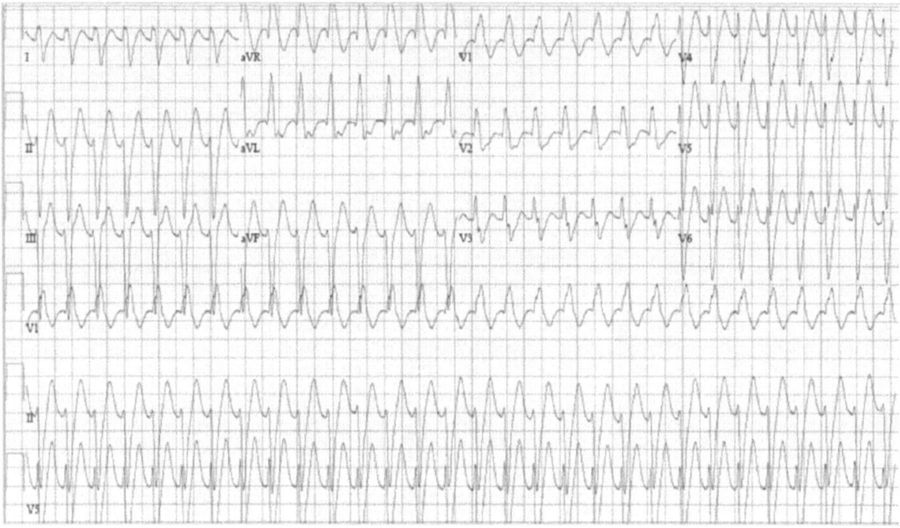

FIGURE 9.70

Rhythm: Supraventricular tachycardia (SVT) [Short-RP tachycardia] with right bundle branch block (RBBB) aberrancy
Rate: 180 BPM
Axis: Northwestern axis deviation
Intervals: Normal
P-wave: Not applicable
QRS Complex: Right bundle branch block (RBBB)
T-wave: T-wave inversions (TWIs) and ST-segment depressions (STDs) in Leads aVL, V2, and V3
Infarct: None

This ECG demonstrates a wide-complex tachycardia with a right bundle branch block (RBBB) morphology. By Brugada criteria, the patient does have RS-waves, and the R-S nadir is <80 ms. Moreover, there is no evidence of atrioventricular (AV) dissociation, and the RBBB has a typical morphology in Lead V1. The rSR' in Lead V1 is typical, as the r-wave is smaller in amplitude than the R'-wave. Although the RBBB morphology in Lead V6 is atypical, morphological criteria for VT are not met, and as such, this tracing represents a supraventricular tachycardia (SVT) with RBBB aberrancy. The QRS axis on this tracing is a Northwestern axis (also known as an extreme right axis, or a superior axis), due to the S-waves in both Leads I and II being greater in amplitude than their respective R-waves. There are T-wave inversions (TWIs) and ST-segment depressions (STDs) in Leads aVL, V2, and V3, which may be related to coronary hypoperfusion due to the rapid heart rate (HR), rather than ischemia.

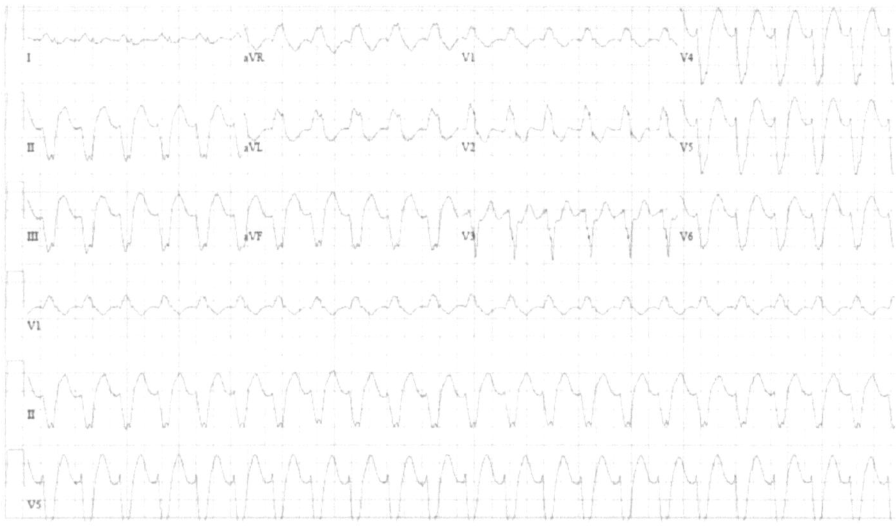

FIGURE 9.71

Rhythm: Ventricular tachycardia (VT) with right bundle branch block morphology
Rate: 138 BPM
Axis: Left axis deviation (LAD)
Intervals: Normal
P-wave: Not applicable
QRS Complex: Right bundle branch block (RBBB)
T-wave: Not applicable
Infarct: None

This ECG demonstrates a wide-complex tachycardia with a right bundle branch block (RBBB) morphology. By Brugada criteria, the patient does have RS-waves, and the R-S nadir is >80 ms. There is no evidence of atrioventricular (AV) dissociation, but the RBBB has an atypical morphology in Leads V1 and V6. The RSr' in Lead V1 is atypical, as the R-wave is larger in amplitude than the r'-wave. The presence of an rS complex (r-wave amplitude < S-wave amplitude) in Lead V6 also favors ventricular tachycardia (VT). There is a left axis deviation (LAD) present in this ECG as well, as indicated by the R-wave amplitude > S-wave amplitude in Lead I, in contrast to the R-wave amplitude < S-wave amplitude in Lead II.

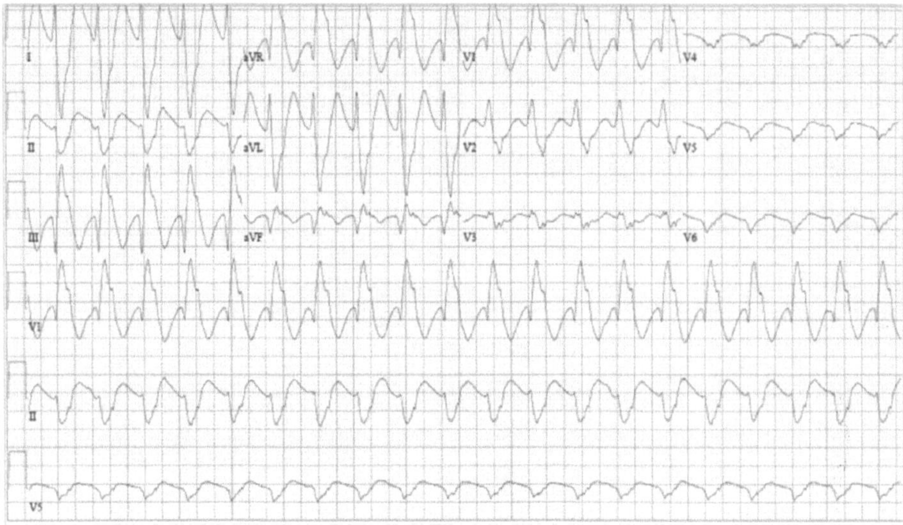

FIGURE 9.72

Rhythm: Ventricular tachycardia (VT) with right bundle branch block morphology
Rate: 120 BPM
Axis: Northwestern axis deviation
Intervals: Normal
P-wave: Not applicable
QRS Complex: Right bundle branch block (RBBB)
T-wave: Not applicable
Infarct: None

This ECG demonstrates a wide-complex tachycardia with a right bundle branch block (RBBB) morphology. By Brugada criteria, the patient does have RS-waves, and the R-S nadir is >80 ms. There is no evidence of atrioventricular (AV) dissociation, but the RBBB has an atypical morphology in Leads V1 and V6. The RSr' in Lead V1 is atypical, as the R-wave is larger in amplitude than the r'-wave. The presence of a monophasic S-wave (r-wave amplitude < S-wave amplitude) in Lead V6 also favors ventricular tachycardia (VT). The QRS axis on this tracing is a Northwestern axis (also known as an extreme right axis, or a superior axis), due to the S-waves in both Leads I and II being greater in amplitude than their respective R-waves.

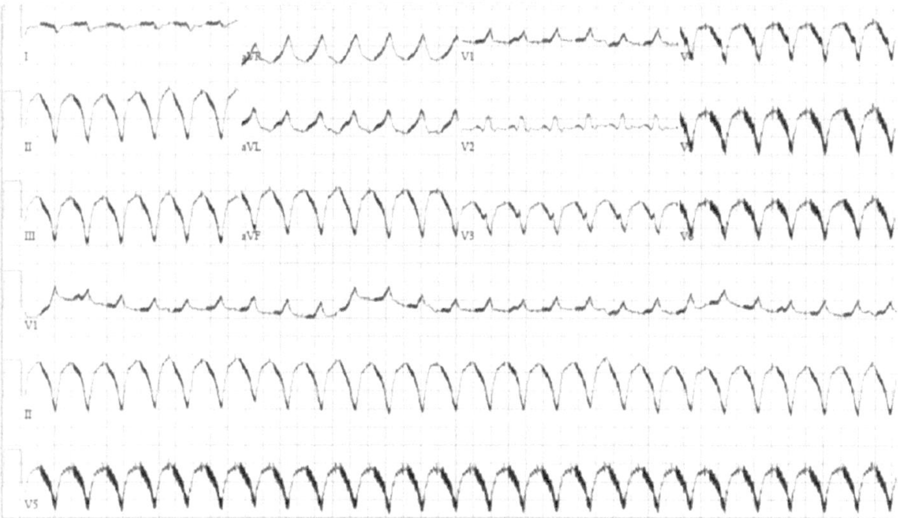

FIGURE 9.73

Rhythm: Ventricular tachycardia (VT) with right bundle branch block morphology
Rate: 156 BPM
Axis: Northwestern axis deviation
Intervals: Normal
P-wave: Not applicable
QRS Complex: Right bundle branch block (RBBB)
T-wave: Not applicable
Infarct: None

This ECG demonstrates a wide-complex tachycardia with a right bundle branch block (RBBB) morphology. By Brugada criteria, the patient does not have RS-waves, which immediately favors ventricular tachycardia (VT). There is no evidence of atrioventricular (AV) dissociation, but the RBBB has an atypical morphology in Leads V1 and V6. The RBBB in Lead V1 is atypical, as there is a monophasic R-wave. The presence of a monophasic S-wave in Lead V6 also favors (VT). By aVR criteria, the patient has a dominant, initial R-wave, another hallmark of VT. This tracing displays Josephson's sign, which is a notching on the downstroke of the S-wave; this is best appreciated in Lead V3, and is another finding consistent with VT. The QRS axis on this tracing is a Northwestern axis (also known as an extreme right axis, or a superior axis), due to the S-waves in both Leads I and II being greater in amplitude than their respective R-waves. Finally, this patient is a recipient of a left ventricular assist device (LVAD), which explains the thickness of the lines in this tracing. The "hum" of the LVAD registers on the ECG leads, causing the above artifact.

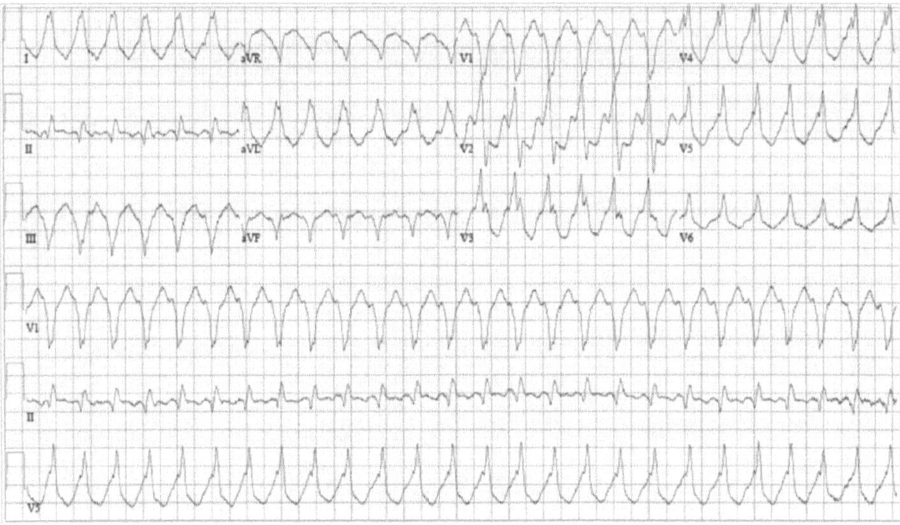

FIGURE 9.74

Rhythm: Ventricular tachycardia (VT) with left bundle branch block morphology
Rate: 156 BPM
Axis: Normal (Physiologic)
Intervals: Normal
P-wave: Not applicable
QRS Complex: Left bundle branch block (LBBB)
T-wave: Not applicable
Infarct: None

This ECG demonstrates a wide-complex tachycardia with a left bundle branch block (LBBB) morphology. By Brugada criteria, the patient does have RS-waves, and the R-S nadir is >80 ms. There is no evidence of atrioventricular (AV) dissociation, and although Leads V1 and V6 have typical morphologies, the R-S nadir duration rules this tracing in for ventricular tachycardia (VT). By aVR criteria, the patient has a Q-wave >40 ms, with an associated notch on the downstroke, another hallmark of VT.

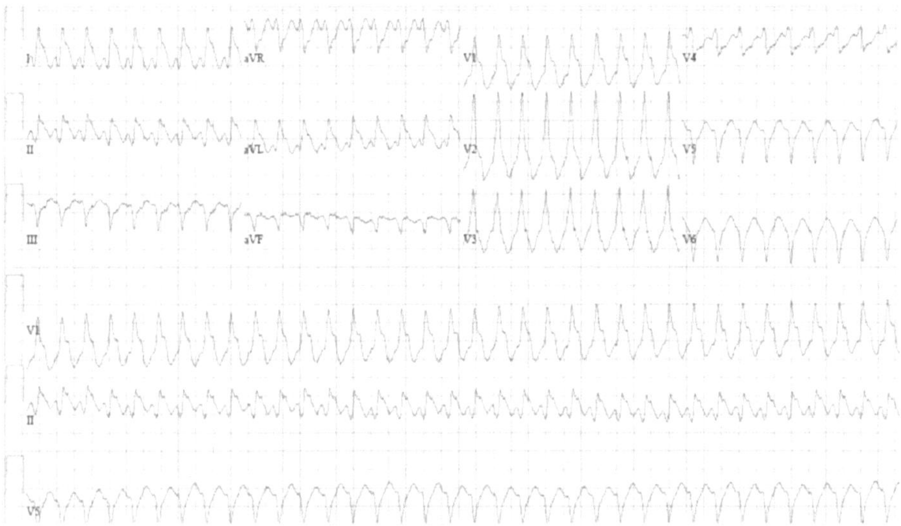

FIGURE 9.75

Rhythm: Ventricular tachycardia (VT) with right bundle branch block morphology
Rate: 216 BPM
Axis: Normal (Physiologic)
Intervals: Normal
P-wave: Not applicable
QRS Complex: Right bundle branch block (RBBB)
T-wave: Not applicable
Infarct: None

This ECG demonstrates a wide-complex tachycardia with a right bundle branch block (RBBB) morphology. By Brugada criteria, the patient does have RS-waves, and the R-S nadir is >80 ms. The intermittent presence of a small, positive deflection in the upstroke of the R-wave, best appreciated in Lead V1, may be evidence of atrioventricular (AV) dissociation. Additionally, the RBBB in Lead V1 is atypical, as there is an RSr'-wave. The presence of a monophasic S-wave in Lead V6 also favors ventricular tachycardia (VT). By aVR criteria, the patient has an initial R-wave >40 ms in duration, another hallmark of VT.

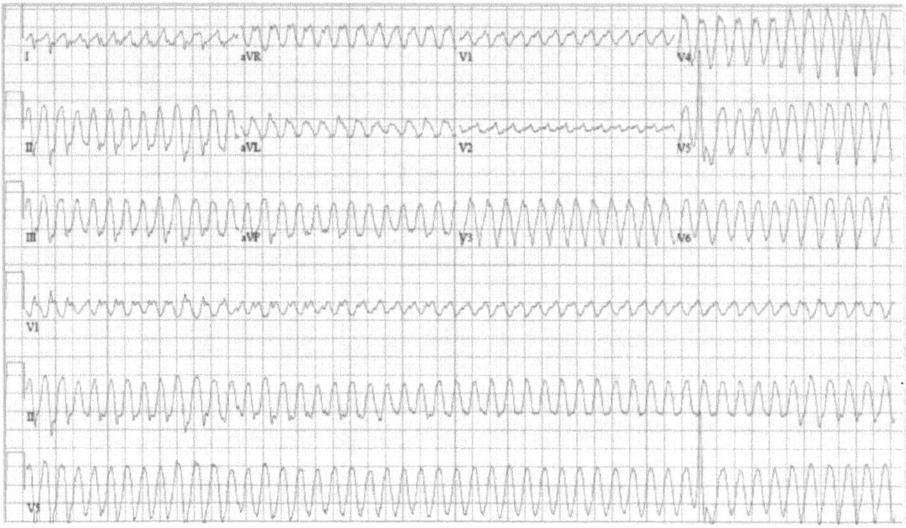

FIGURE 9.76

Rhythm: Ventricular flutter
Rate: 300 BPM
Axis: Not applicable
Intervals: Normal
P-wave: Not applicable
QRS Complex: Not applicable
T-wave: Not applicable
Infarct: Not applicable

This ECG demonstrates a wide complex tachycardia, but unlike supraventricular tachycardia (SVT) with aberrancy or ventricular tachycardia (VT), the architecture of the QRS is lost. Namely, there is a loss of P-waves, QRS complexes, and T-waves. A wide complex tachycardia with this morphology, particularly at a rate around 300 BPM, is consistent with ventricular flutter. Ventricular flutter is the harbinger of circulatory collapse and cardiopulmonary arrest. This rhythm typically degenerates into ventricular fibrillation (VF). The abnormal beat noted in Lead V5 is an artifact, as the same abnormality is not noted in any other Lead.

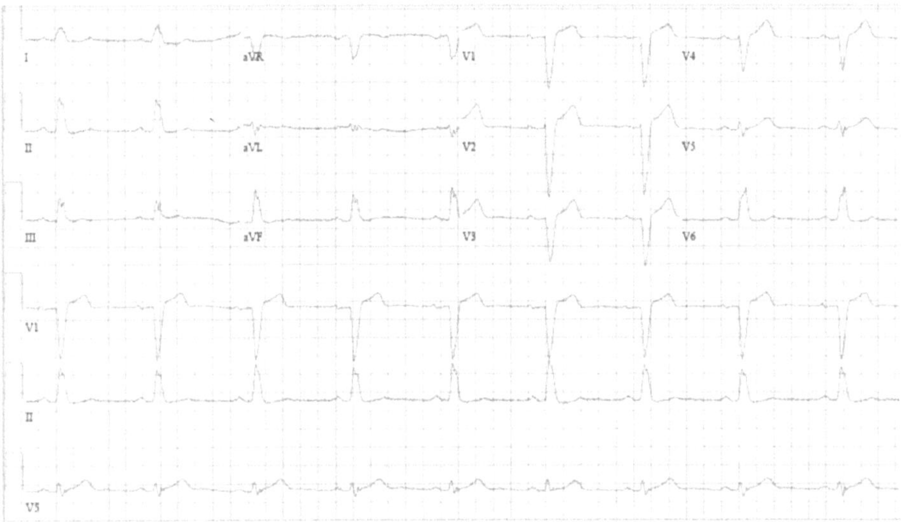

FIGURE 9.77

Rhythm: Sinus bradycardia
Rate: 57 BPM
Axis: Normal (Physiologic)
Intervals: QRS complex duration >120 ms
P-wave: Normal
QRS Complex: Left bundle branch block (LBBB)
T-wave: Repolarization abnormalities from LBBB
Infarct: None

This ECG demonstrates normal sinus rhythm (NSR), as the P-waves in Leads I, II, and aVF are positive, and the P-wave in Lead V1 is biphasic. Also present is a left bundle branch block (LBBB) (best appreciated in Leads V1, V2, and V6) with a typical rS-wave in Lead V1, a monophasic R-wave in Lead V6, and a total QRS complex duration of >120 ms. There are associated repolarization abnormalities in Leads V1–V3, and V6 from the LBBB.

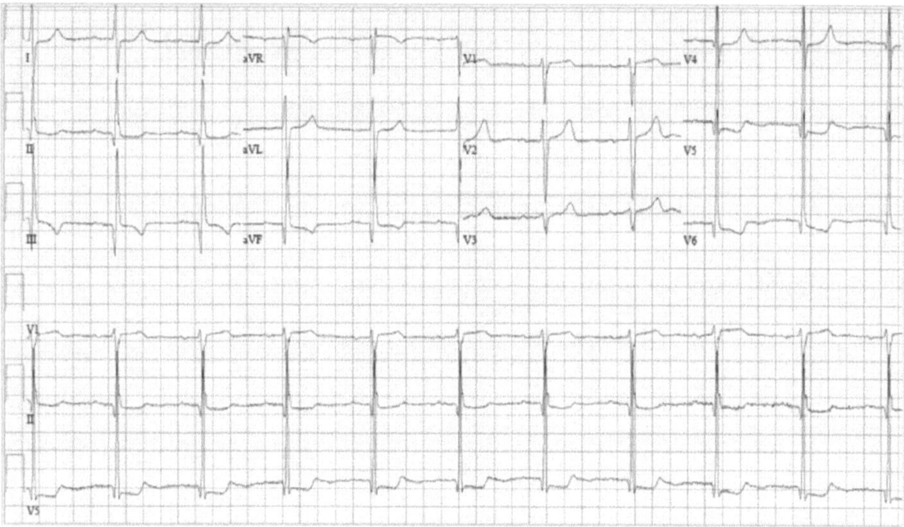

FIGURE 9.78

Rhythm: Sinus rhythm
Rate: 66 BPM
Axis: Normal (Physiologic)
Intervals: Normal
P-wave: P-wave flattening
QRS Complex: Left ventricular hypertrophy (LVH)
T-wave: Diffuse repolarization abnormalities
Infarct: None

This ECG demonstrates normal sinus rhythm (NSR), as the P-waves in Leads I, II, and aVF are positive, and the P-wave in Lead V1 is biphasic. There is nonspecific flattening of the P-waves. Based upon the Sokolow–Lyon criteria—namely the sum of the mV in V1S and V5R—left ventricular hypertrophy (LVH) is present. The diffuse repolarization abnormalities—namely, ST-segment depressions (STDs)—are a consequence of the LVH.

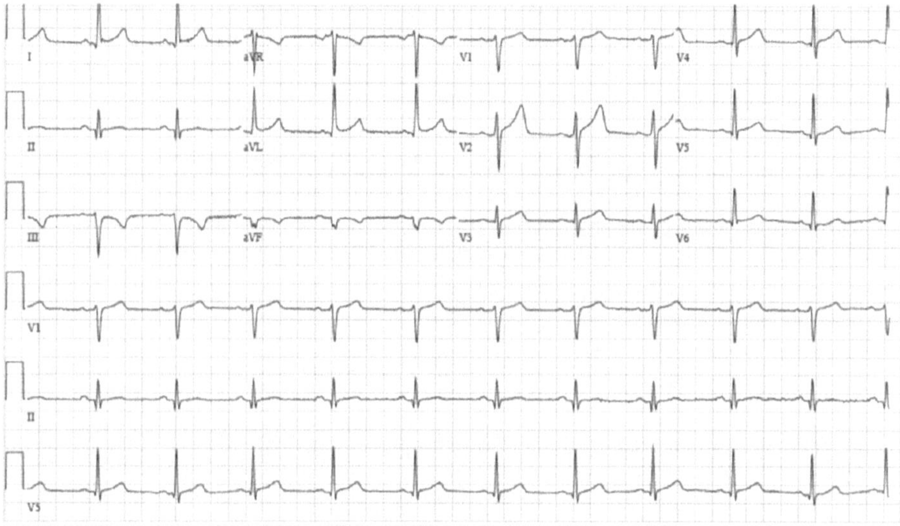

FIGURE 9.79

Rhythm: Sinus rhythm
Rate: 68 BPM
Axis: Normal (Physiologic)
Intervals: Normal
P-wave: Normal
QRS Complex: Left ventricular hypertrophy (LVH)
T-wave: T-wave inversions (TWIs) and T-wave flattening in Leads II, III, and aVF
Infarct: Prior Inferior Wall Infarction

This ECG demonstrates normal sinus rhythm (NSR), as the P-waves in Leads I, II, and aVF are positive. Based upon the modified Cornell criteria, the R-wave >11 mm in amplitude in Lead aVL is suggestive of left ventricular hypertrophy (LVH), although a similar pattern may exist as a normal variant. T-wave inversions (TWIs) are present along Leads III and aVF, along with nonspecific T-wave flattening in Lead II. Based upon the q-waves in Leads II, III, and aVF, there is evidence of a prior inferior wall myocardial infarction.

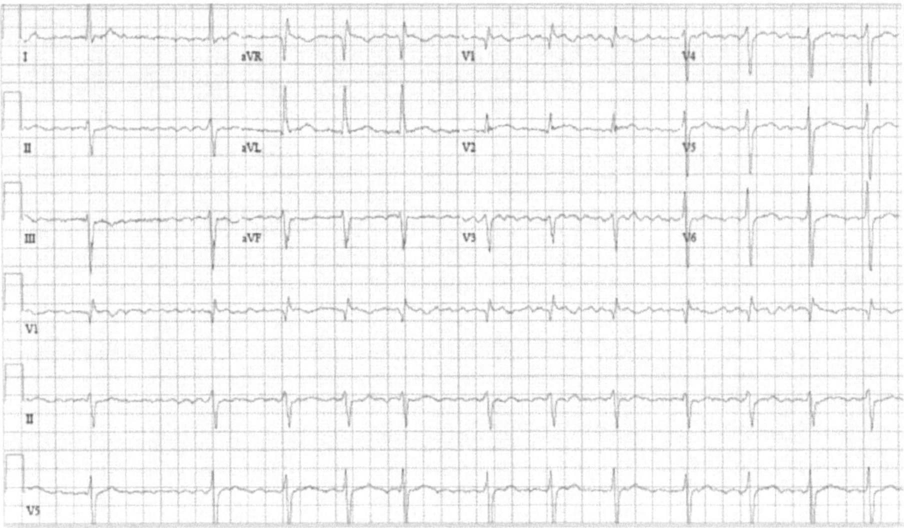

FIGURE 9.80

Rhythm: Atrial fibrillation with a controlled ventricular response (CVR)
Rate: 70 BPM
Axis: Left axis deviation (LAD)
Intervals: Normal
P-wave: Not applicable
QRS Complex: Left ventricular hypertrophy (LVH)
T-wave: None
Infarct: None

This ECG demonstrates a lack of discernable P-waves amidst a random oscillation of electrical activity along the baseline, which is consistent with atrial fibrillation (Afib). The f-waves (fibrillatory waves) are characterized by random deflections that vary in terms of duration, amplitude, and morphology. This is associated with an irregularly irregular RR interval with a controlled ventricular response (CVR), due to the ventricular heart rate between 60 BPM and 100 BPM. There is a left axis deviation (LAD) present in this ECG as well, as indicated by the R-wave amplitude > S-wave amplitude in Lead I, in contrast to the R-wave amplitude < S-wave amplitude in Lead II. Based upon the modified Cornell criteria, the R-wave >11 mm in amplitude in Lead aVL is indicative of left ventricular hypertrophy (LVH).

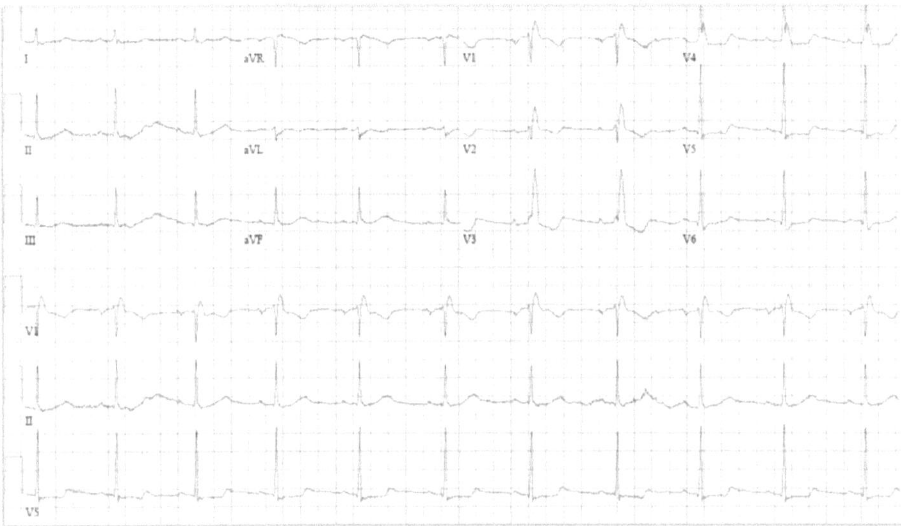

FIGURE 9.81

Rhythm: Sinus rhythm
Rate: 69 BPM
Axis: Normal (Physiologic)
Intervals: Normal
P-wave: Normal
QRS Complex: Right bundle branch block (RBBB)
T-wave: Diffuse repolarization abnormalities
Infarct: None

This ECG demonstrates normal sinus rhythm (NSR), as the P-waves in Leads I, II, and aVF are positive, and the P-wave in Lead V1 is biphasic. An rSR' is present in Lead V1, and the QRS complex is >120 ms in duration, which is consistent with a right bundle branch block (RBBB). There are diffuse repolarization abnormalities, namely ST-segment depressions (STDs) and corresponding T-wave inversions (TWIs) that may be a consequence of the RBBB. However, the ST-segment depressions (STDs) in Leads V4–V6 are unlikely to be explained by the RBBB and may represent concomitant ischemia.

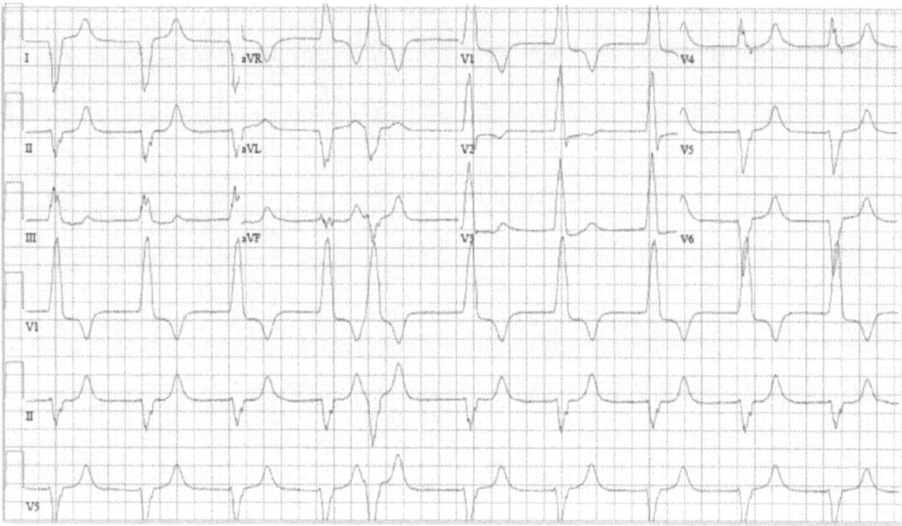

FIGURE 9.82

Rhythm: Idioventricular rhythm
Rate: 60 BPM
Axis: Northwestern axis deviation
Intervals: QTc prolongation >500 ms, QRS complex >120 ms
P-wave: Not applicable
QRS Complex: Right Ventricular Hypertrophy, Reverse R-wave Progression, QRS complex duration >120 ms
T-wave: ST-segment depressions (STDs) in Leads III, aVF, V2, and V3
Infarct: None

This ECG demonstrates an idioventricular rhythm, as the RR interval is regular with possible retrograde P-waves (best appreciated in Lead II) and a wide QRS complex >120 ms in duration. There are ST-segment depressions (STDs) in Leads III, aVF, V2, and V3. The tall R-waves along Leads V1–V4 in conjunction with the aforementioned repolarization abnormalities raise concern for right ventricular hypertrophy (RVH). Additionally, the monophasic R-wave in lead aVR, the monophasic S-wave in Leads I and aVL, and the reverse R-wave progression along the precordial Leads are concerning for dextrocardia. This particular patient had Tetralogy of Fallot (ToF) and heart failure with a reduced ejection fraction (HFrEF). There is a prolonged QTc interval in this patient, with the QTc measuring around 500 ms. The QRS axis on this tracing is a Northwestern axis (also known as an extreme right axis, or a superior axis), due to the S-waves in both Leads I and II being greater in amplitude than their respective R-waves.

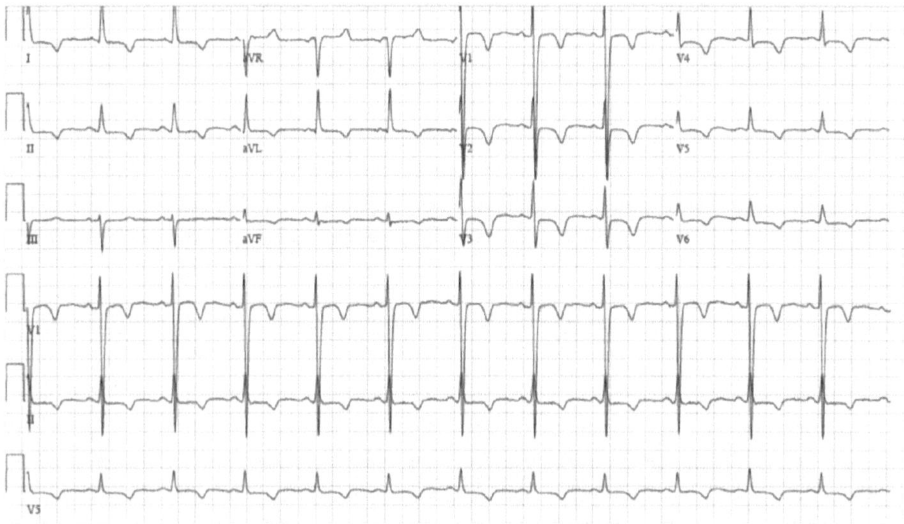

FIGURE 9.83

Rhythm: Sinus rhythm
Rate: 73 BPM
Axis: Normal (Physiologic)
Intervals: QT-interval prolongation >500 ms
P-wave: Normal
QRS Complex: Left and right ventricular hypertrophy
T-wave: Diffuse T-wave inversions (TWIs)
Infarct: None

This ECG demonstrates normal sinus rhythm (NSR), as the P-waves in Leads I, II, and aVF are positive. There are diffuse T-wave inversions (TWIs) along the precordial leads (V1–V6), as well as in Leads I, aVL, II, and aVF. These are accompanied by 1 mm ST-segment depressions (STDs) along Leads V2–V4, as well as in Leads I and II. This tracing would be concerning for ischemia along the anterior, lateral, and inferior walls of the left ventricle (LV). However, other diagnoses, such as increased intracranial pressure or hypertrophic cardiomyopathy could be considered. Based upon the modified Cornell criteria, the R-wave >11 mm in amplitude in Lead aVL is indicative of left ventricular hypertrophy (LVH). The corrected QT-interval (QTc) is prolonged in this tracing, being ~500 ms in duration.

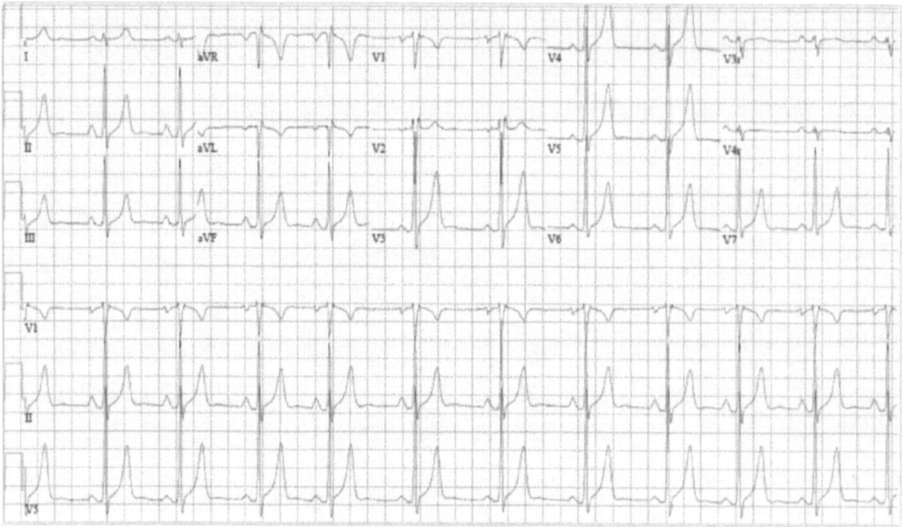

FIGURE 9.84

Rhythm: Sinus rhythm
Rate: 71 BPM
Axis: Normal (Physiological)
Intervals: Normal
P-wave: Normal
QRS Complex: J-point elevation
T-wave: ST-segment elevations in Leads II, III, aVF, and V3–V6
Infarct: None

This ECG demonstrates normal sinus rhythm (NSR), as the P-waves in Leads I, II, and aVF are positive, and the P-wave in Lead V1 is biphasic. There is J-point elevation (also known as early repolarization) evident over the anterior and inferior leads. There are no ST-segment depressions (STDs), T-wave inversions (TWIs), or pathological Q-waves to suggest the ST-segment elevations (STEs) in Leads II, III, aVF, and V3–V6 are related to ischemia or infarction.

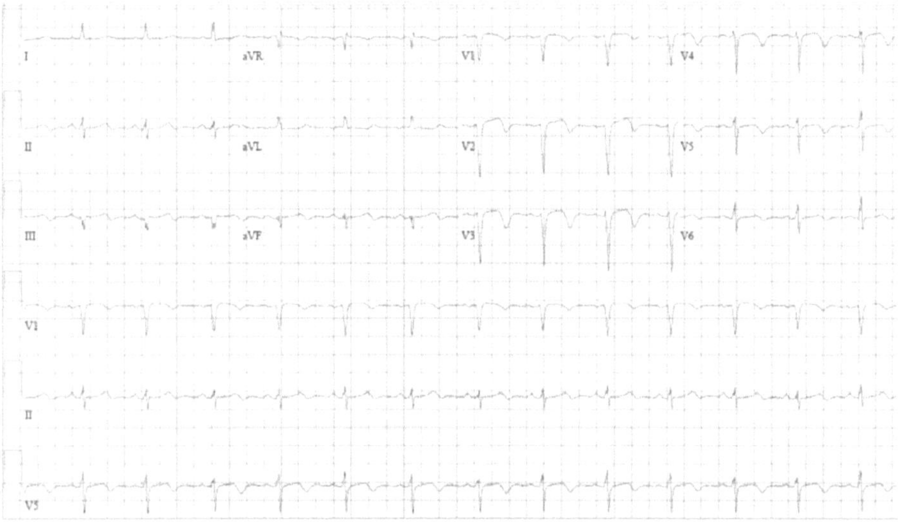

FIGURE 9.85

Rhythm: Sinus rhythm
Rate: 80 BPM
Axis: Left axis deviation (LAD)
Intervals: Normal
P-wave: Normal
QRS Complex: Poor R-wave progression (PRWP)
T-wave: Biphasic anterior T-wave inversions (TWIs)
Infarct: None

This ECG demonstrates normal sinus rhythm (NSR), as the P-waves in Leads I, II, and aVF are positive, and the P-wave in Lead V1 is biphasic. There is a left axis deviation (LAD) present in this ECG as well, as indicated by the R-wave amplitude > S-wave amplitude in Lead I, in contrast to the R-wave amplitude < S-wave amplitude in Lead II. There are biphasic T-wave inversions (TWIs) present along the anterior Leads, although the biphasic T-waves are most notable over leads V1–V3. There is concomitant poor R-wave progression (PRWP) along the anterior Leads. Taken together, these findings are concerning for Wellens' T-waves (specifically the Type A pattern). Clinically, this would be indicative of critical left anterior descending artery stenosis.

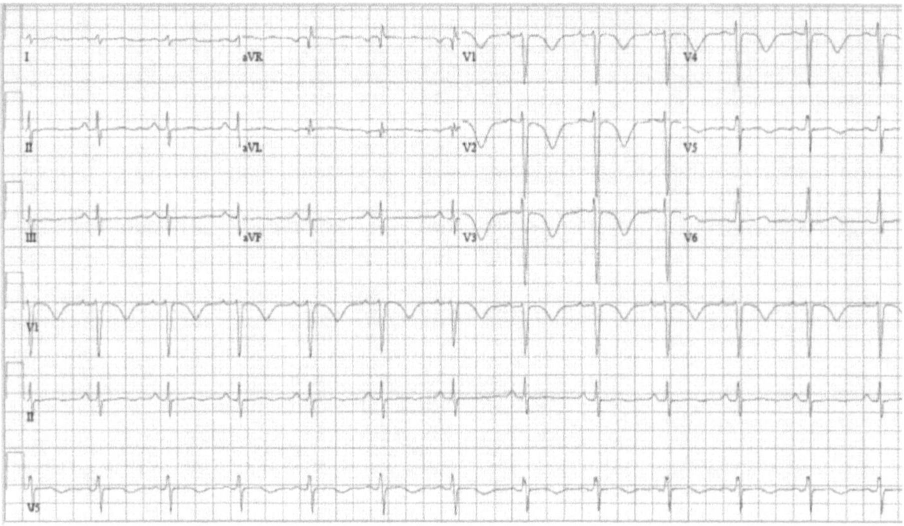

FIGURE 9.86

Rhythm: Sinus rhythm
Rate: 68 BPM
Axis: Normal (Physiological)
Intervals: Normal
P-wave: Normal
QRS Complex: Poor R-wave progression (PRWP)
T-wave: Monophasic anterior T-wave inversions (TWIs)
Infarct: None

This ECG demonstrates normal sinus rhythm (NSR), as the P-waves in Leads I, II, and aVF are positive, and the P-wave in Lead V1 is biphasic. There are monophasic T-wave inversions (TWIs) present along the anterior Leads, although the monophasic TWIs are most notable over leads V1–V4. There is concomitant poor R-wave progression (PRWP) along the anterior Leads. Taken together, these findings are concerning for Wellens' T-waves (specifically the Type B pattern). Clinically, this would be indicative of critical left anterior descending artery stenosis. However, other clinical vignettes, such as an acute intracranial process, can produce similar ECG patterns; as such, integrations of the ECG findings with the clinic vignette are necessary for proper interpretation.

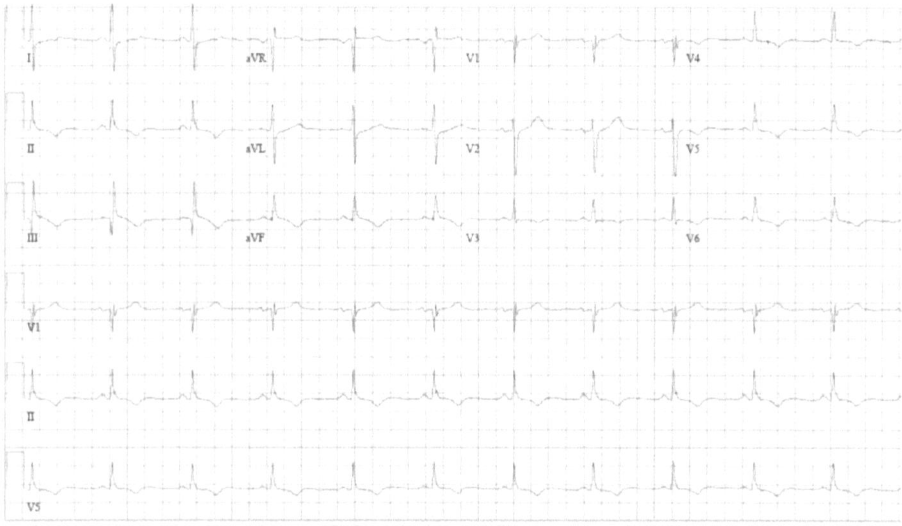

FIGURE 9.87

Rhythm: Sinus rhythm
Rate: 67 BPM
Axis: Normal (Physiological)
Intervals: Normal
P-wave: Normal
QRS Complex: Normal
T-wave: T-wave inversions (TWIs) and ST-segment depression (STDs) in Leads II, III, aVF, and V3–V6.
Infarct: None

This ECG demonstrates normal sinus rhythm (NSR), as the P-waves in Leads I, II, and aVF are positive, and the P-wave in Lead V1 is biphasic. There are T-wave inversions (TWIs) and ST-segment depressions (STDs) along Leads II, III, aVF, and V3–V6, concerning for inferolateral ischemia.

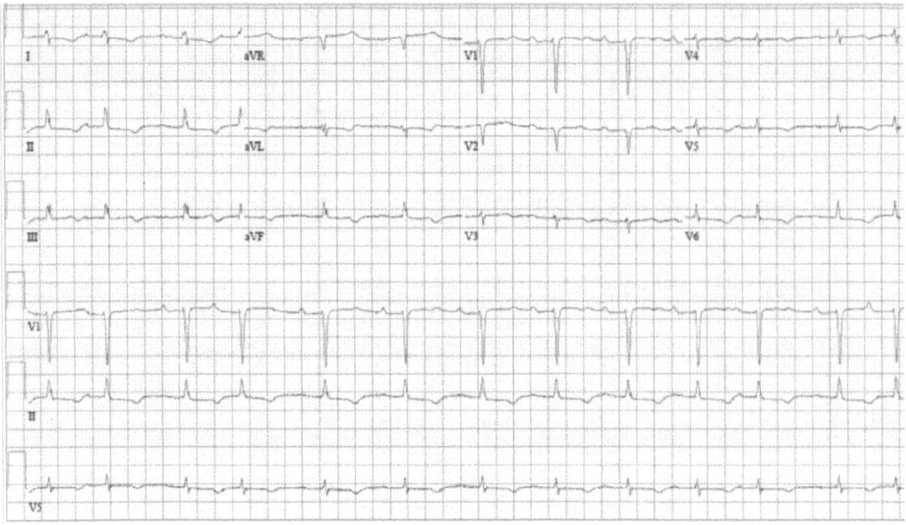

FIGURE 9.88

Rhythm: Sinus rhythm
Rate: 77 BPM
Axis: Normal (Physiological)
Intervals: Normal
P-wave: Normal
QRS Complex: Normal
T-wave: T-wave inversions (TWIs) and ST-segment depression (STDs) in Leads I, II, III, aVF, aVL, and V3–V6.
Infarct: Pathological Q-waves in V1 and V2, Septal myocardial infarction (MI)

This ECG demonstrates normal sinus rhythm (NSR), as the P-waves in Leads I, II, and aVF are positive, and the P-wave in Lead V1 is biphasic. There are T-wave inversions (TWIs) and ST-segment depressions (STDs) along Leads I, II, III, aVF, aVL, and V3–V6, concerning for inferolateral ischemia. There are pathological Q-waves along the anteroseptal Leads (V1 and V2), which were likely due to a septal myocardial infarction (MI). The 2nd and 4th beats on the rhythm strip are premature atrial contractions (PACs).

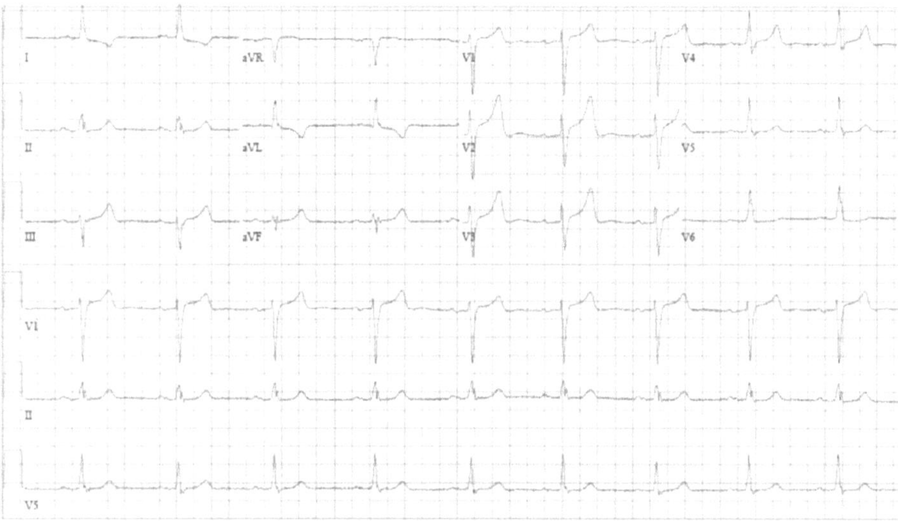

FIGURE 9.89

Rhythm: Sinus bradycardia
Rate: 58 BPM
Axis: Normal (Physiological)
Intervals: PR interval >200 ms (1st Degree AV delay)
P-wave: Normal
QRS Complex: Normal
T-wave: T-wave inversions (TWIs) and ST-segment depression (STDs) in Leads I, aVL, and V6; Early repolarization
Infarct: None

This ECG demonstrates normal sinus rhythm (NSR), as the P-waves in Leads I, II, and aVF are positive, and the P-wave in Lead V1 is biphasic. The PR interval is >200 ms, which is indicative of a 1st degree atrioventricular (AV) delay. The ST-segment elevations (STEs) in Leads V1–V4 represent J-point elevation (also known as early repolarization), which was present on previous ECGs for this particular patient. There are T-wave inversions (TWIs) and ST-segment depressions (STDs) along Leads I, aVL, and V6, concerning for lateral ischemia.

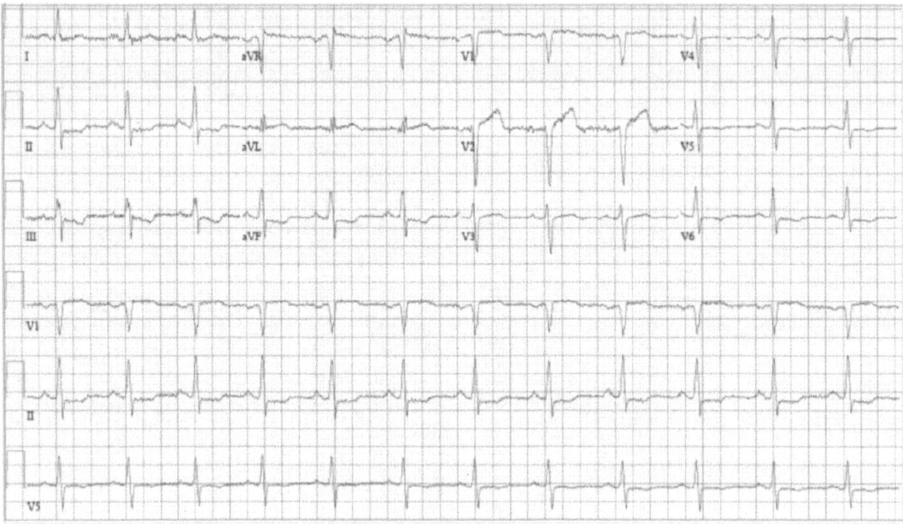

FIGURE 9.90

Rhythm: Sinus rhythm
Rate: 71 BPM
Axis: Normal (Physiological)
Intervals: Normal
P-wave: Normal
QRS Complex: Poor R-wave progression (PRWP)
T-wave: T-wave inversions (TWIs) and ST-segment depression (STDs) in Leads II, III, aVF, V5, and V6
Infarct: Pathological septal Q-waves, Septal myocardial infarction (MI), Left ventricular (LV) aneurysm in Lead V2

This ECG demonstrates normal sinus rhythm (NSR), as the P-waves in Leads I, II, and aVF are positive, and the P-wave in Lead V1 is biphasic. There are T-wave inversions (TWIs) and ST-segment depressions (STDs) along Leads II, III, aVF, V5, and V6, concerning for ischemia. Additionally, there are pathological Q-waves along the septal Leads (V1 and V2), which were likely due to a septal myocardial infarction (MI). Furthermore, there is evidence of a left ventricular (LV) aneurysm due to a persistent ST-segment elevation (STE) in Lead V2. There is concomitant poor R-wave progression (PRWP) along the anterior Leads, as the QRS complex does not become predominantly positive until Lead V5.

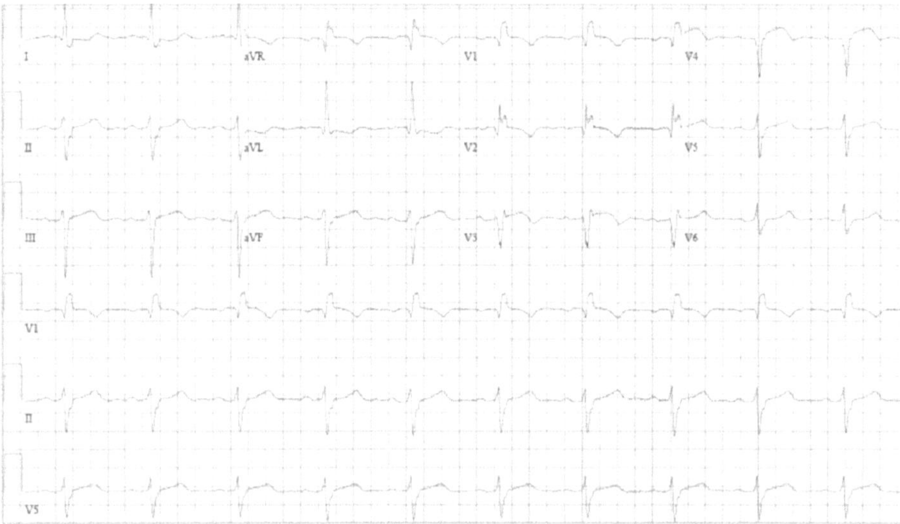

FIGURE 9.91

Rhythm: Sinus rhythm
Rate: 61 BPM
Axis: Left axis deviation (LAD)
Intervals: PR interval >200 ms (1st Degree AV delay)
P-wave: Normal
QRS Complex: Right bundle branch block (RBBB)
T-wave: ST-segment elevations (STEs) in Leads V3–V5, T-wave inversions (TWIs) and ST-segment depression (STDs) in Leads I and aVL
Infarct: Pathological Q-waves in Leads V1–V4, Anterolateral myocardial infarction (MI)

This ECG demonstrates normal sinus rhythm (NSR), as the P-waves in Leads I, II, and aVF are positive, and the P-wave in Lead V1 is biphasic. The PR interval is >200 ms, which is indicative of a 1st degree atrioventricular (AV) delay. The ST-segment elevations (STEs) in Leads V3–V5 represent an anterolateral ST-segment elevation myocardial infarction (STEMI). Additionally, there are already pathological Q-waves in Leads V1–V4, indicating a later presentation to the hospital. There are reciprocal T-wave inversions (TWIs) and ST-segment depressions (STDs) along Leads I and aVL. An rSR' is present in Lead V1, and the QRS complex is >120 ms in duration, which is consistent with a right bundle branch block (RBBB). There is a left axis deviation (LAD) present in this ECG as well, as indicated by the R-wave amplitude > S-wave amplitude in Lead I, in contrast to the R-wave amplitude < S-wave amplitude in Lead II.

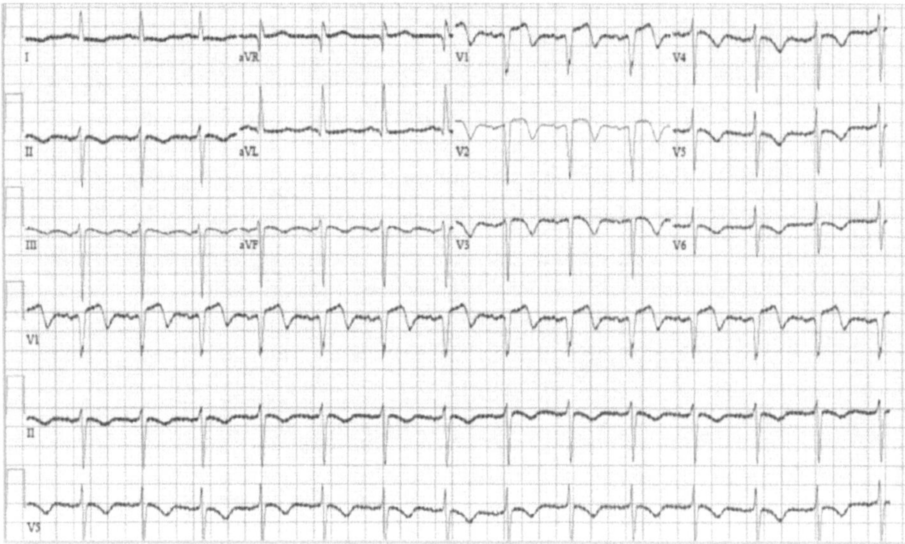

FIGURE 9.92

Rhythm: Ectopic atrial rhythm with anteroseptal STEMI
Rate: 86 BPM
Axis: Left axis deviation (LAD)
Intervals: ST-segment elevation (STE) in V1–V3
P-wave: Ectopic
QRS Complex: Pathological Q-waves in V1–V3; Poor R-wave progression (PRWP); Left anterior hemiblock (LAH)
T-wave: T-wave inversions (TWIs) in V1–V6, and Leads II, III, and aVF
Infarct: Acute anteroseptal ST-segment elevation myocardial infarction (STEMI)

This ECG is most concerning for a late-presenting anterior wall STEMI, which is corroborated by 3–4 mm ST-segment elevations (STEs) in Leads V1–V3. These STEs are associated with wide (>40 ms in duration) pathological Q-waves along the same territory, along with T-wave inversions (TWIs) in Leads V1–V6, II, III, and aVF. Additionally, this tracing has a regular RR interval but is not indicative of sinus rhythm. The P-waves within Leads II, III, and aVF are inverted (negative amplitude) and, as such, cannot be originating from the sinoatrial (SA) node. This pattern is most consistent with an ectopic atrial rhythm. There is a left axis deviation (LAD) present in this ECG as well, as indicated by the R-wave amplitude > S-wave amplitude in Lead I, in contrast to the R-wave amplitude < S-wave amplitude in Lead II. Additionally, there is a qR-wave present in Leads I and aVL, an rS-wave in Lead III, and a QRS complex that is between 80 ms and 100 ms in duration. This pattern is demonstrative of a left anterior fascicular block (LAFB), which is also known as a left anterior hemiblock (LAH). The LAH explains the LAD in this tracing.

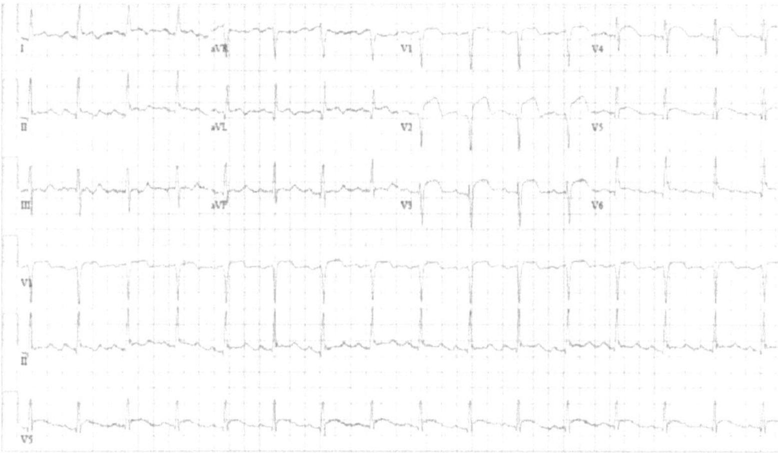

FIGURE 9.93

Rhythm: Sinus rhythm
Rate: 95 BPM
Axis: Normal (Physiological)
Intervals: Normal
P-wave: Normal
QRS Complex: Normal
T-wave: ST-segment elevations (STEs) in Leads I, aVL, V1–V6, T-wave inversions (TWIs) and ST-segment depressions (STDs) in Leads II, III, and aVF
Infarct: Pathological Q-waves in Leads V1 and V2, Anterolateral myocardial infarction (MI)

This ECG demonstrates normal sinus rhythm (NSR), as the P-waves in Leads I, II, and aVF are positive, and the P-wave in Lead V1 is biphasic. The ST-segment elevations (STEs) in Leads I, aVL, and V1–V6 represent an anterolateral ST-segment elevation myocardial infarction (STEMI). Additionally, there are already pathological Q-waves in Leads V1 and V2, indicating a later presentation to the hospital. There are reciprocal T-wave inversions (TWIs) and ST-segment depressions (STDs) along Leads II, III, and aVF.

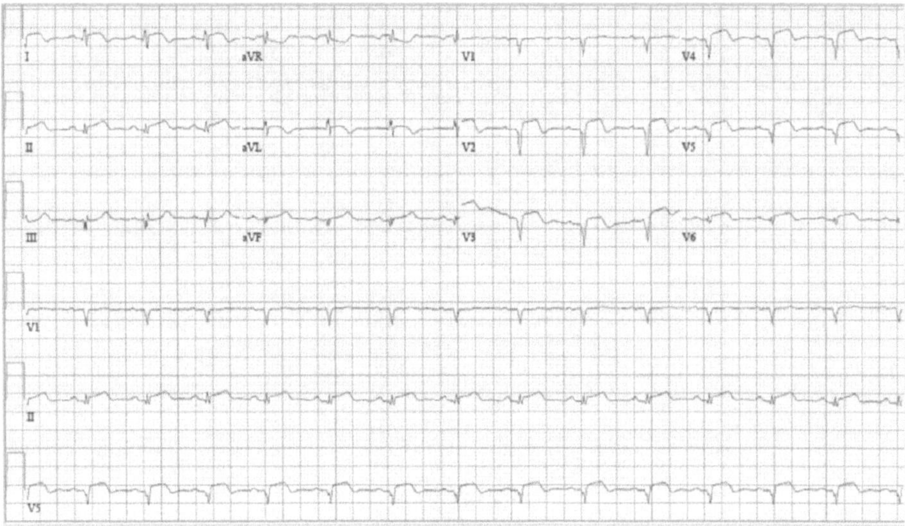

FIGURE 9.94

Rhythm: Sinus rhythm
Rate: 89 BPM
Axis: Right axis deviation (RAD)
Intervals: Normal
P-wave: Normal
QRS Complex: Low voltage
T-wave: ST-segment elevations (STEs) in Leads I, II, aVL, V1–V6, T-wave inversions (TWIs) and ST-segment depressions (STDs) in Lead aVR
Infarct: Pathological Q-waves in Leads V1–V6, Anterolateral myocardial infarction (MI)

This ECG demonstrates normal sinus rhythm (NSR), as the P-waves in Leads I, II, and aVF are positive, and the P-wave in Lead V1 is biphasic. The ST-segment elevations (STEs) in Leads I, II, aVL, and V1–V6 represent an anterolateral ST-segment elevation myocardial infarction (STEMI). Additionally, there are already pathological Q-waves in Leads V1–V6, indicating a late presentation to the hospital. There is a reciprocal T-wave inversion (TWI) and ST-segment depression (STD) along Lead aVR. Furthermore, a right axis deviation (RAD) is present, as the S-wave in Lead I is greater in amplitude than the corresponding R-wave, while the QRS complex in Lead II is positive in polarity. Additionally, QRS complexes <5 mm in amplitude throughout the limb leads are consistent with low voltage.

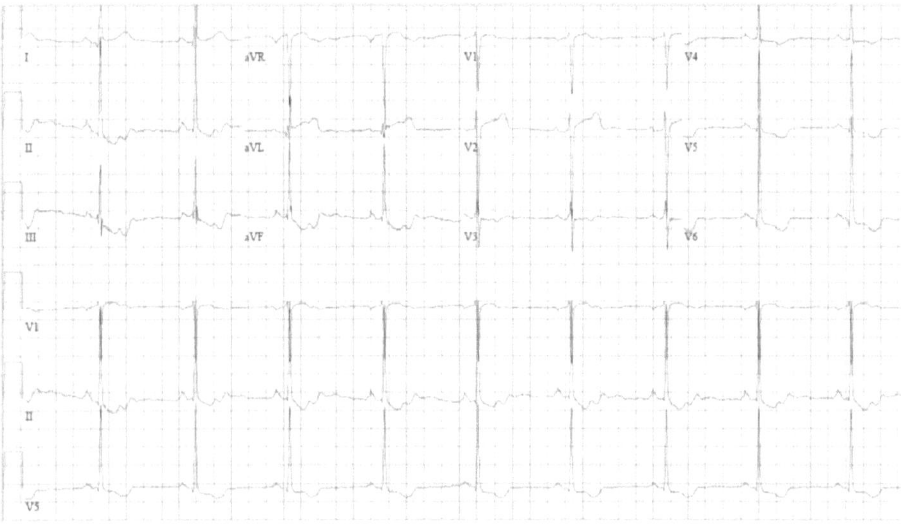

FIGURE 9.95

Rhythm: Sinus bradycardia
Rate: 56 BPM
Axis: Normal (Physiological)
Intervals: Normal
P-wave: Normal
QRS Complex: Left ventricular hypertrophy (LVH)
T-wave: ST-segment elevations (STEs) in Leads I and aVL, T-wave inversions (TWIs) and ST-segment depressions (STDs) in Leads II, III, aVF, V5, and V6
Infarct: Pathological Q-waves in Leads I and aVL

This ECG demonstrates normal sinus rhythm (NSR), as the P-waves in Leads I, II, and aVF are positive, and the P-wave in Lead V1 is biphasic. The ST-segment elevations (STEs) in Leads I and aVL represent a lateral ST-segment elevation myocardial infarction (STEMI). Additionally, there are small pathological Q-waves in Leads I and aVL. There are reciprocal T-wave inversions (TWIs) and ST-segment depressions (STDs) along Leads II, III, aVF, V5, and V6. Based upon the Sokolow–Lyon criteria—namely the sum of the mV in V1S and V5R—left ventricular hypertrophy (LVH) is present.

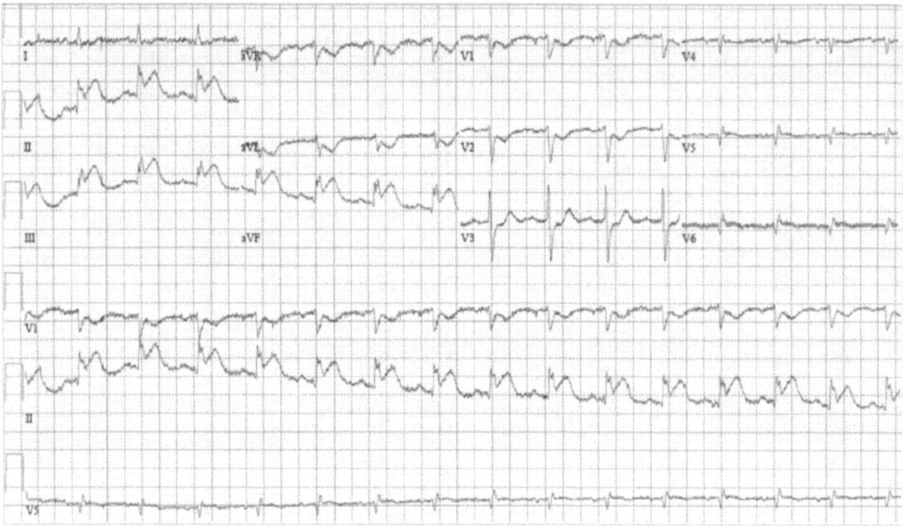

FIGURE 9.96

Rhythm: Sinus rhythm
Rate: 90 BPM
Axis: Normal (Physiological)
Intervals: Normal
P-wave: Normal
QRS Complex: Normal
T-wave: ST-segment elevations (STEs) in Leads II, III, aVF, V5, and V6, T-wave inversions (TWIs) and ST-segment depressions (STDs) in Leads I, aVL, and V1–V3
Infarct: Pathological Q-waves in Leads II, III, and aVF

This ECG demonstrates normal sinus rhythm (NSR), as the P-waves in Leads I, II, and aVF are positive, and the P-wave in Lead V1 is biphasic. The ST-segment elevations (STEs) and small pathological Q-waves in Leads II, III, aVF, V5, and V6 represent an inferior ST-segment elevation myocardial infarction (STEMI). There are reciprocal T-wave inversions (TWIs) and ST-segment depressions (STDs) along Leads I, aVL, and V1–V3. Moreover, the presence of TWI and STD in the anterior leads in the setting of an inferior wall STEMI raises concern for concomitant right ventricular (RV) infarction. The wandering appearance of the Leads is an artifact due to patient movement.

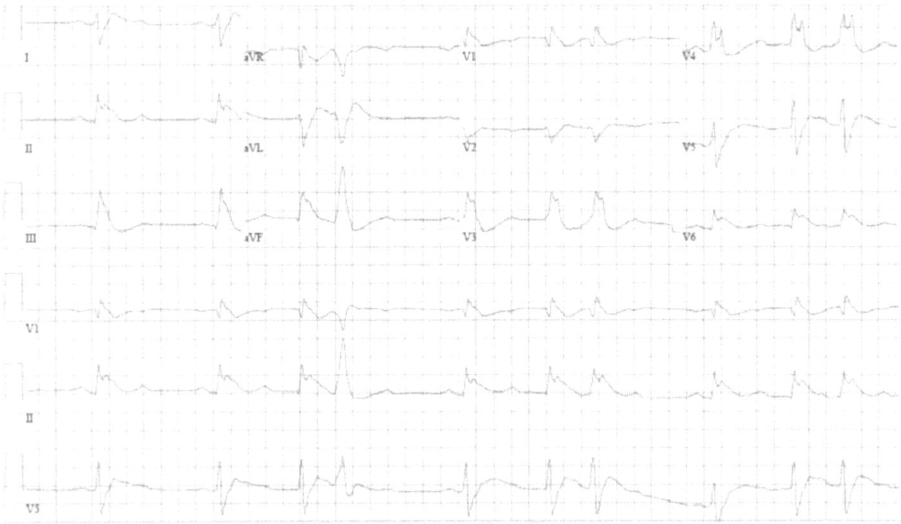

FIGURE 9.97

Rhythm: Sinus rhythm with 3rd Degree atrioventricular (AV) block
Rate: 55 BPM
Axis: Right axis deviation (RAD)
Intervals: Normal
P-wave: Normal
QRS Complex: Myopathic, Right bundle morphology
T-wave: ST-segment elevations (STEs) in Leads II, III, aVF, V5, and V6, T-wave inversions (TWIs) and ST-segment depressions (STDs) in Leads V3 and V4
Infarct: Pathological Q-waves in Leads II, III, and aVF

This ECG demonstrates normal sinus rhythm (NSR), as the P-waves in Leads I, II, and aVF are positive, and the P-wave in Lead V1 is biphasic. The ST-segment elevations (STEs) and small pathological Q-waves in Leads II, III, aVF, V5, and V6 represent an inferior ST-segment elevation myocardial infarction (STEMI). There are reciprocal T-wave inversions (TWIs) and ST-segment depressions (STDs) along Leads V3 and V4. There are P-waves throughout the rhythm strip that do not conduct to an associated QRS complex. However, the PP-interval remains constant throughout the tracing, while the PR-interval varies. The atrial rate (around 80 BPM) is faster than the ventricular rate (paced around 60 BPM); the atria and the ventricles are depolarizing independently of one another. This pattern of AV dissociation in the context of an atrial rate faster than the ventricular rate is consistent with 3rd degree atrioventricular block (AVB), otherwise known as complete heart block (CHB). The myopathic-appearing QRS complex in this tracing, right bundle morphology, and the presence of AV blocks is in the context of acidemia following a cardiac arrest. Finally, a right axis deviation (RAD) is present, as the S-wave in Lead I is greater in amplitude than the corresponding R-wave, while the QRS complex in Leads II and aVF are positive in amplitude.

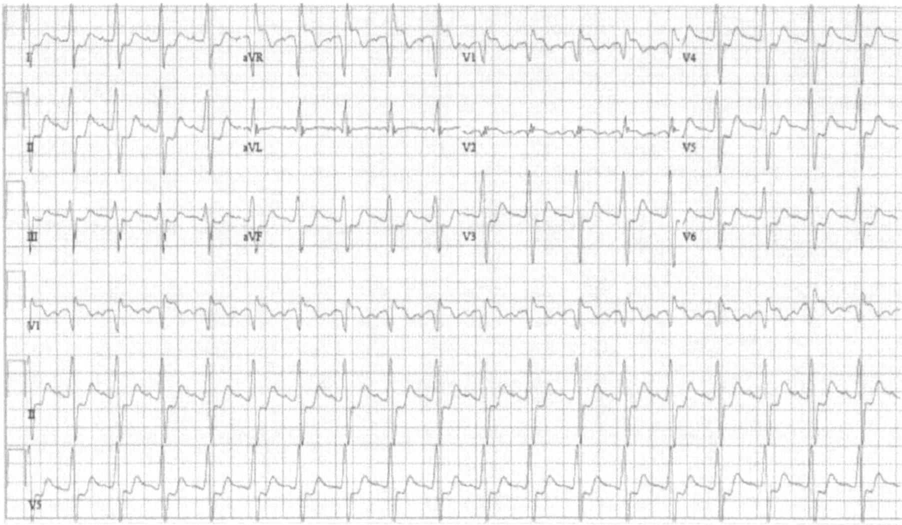

FIGURE 9.98

Rhythm: Sinus tachycardia
Rate: 113 BPM
Axis: Normal (Physiological)
Intervals: Normal
P-wave: Normal
QRS Complex: Right bundle branch block (RBBB)
T-wave: ST-segment elevations (STEs) in Leads aVR, V1, and V2, T-wave inversions (TWIs) and ST-segment depressions (STDs) in Leads I, II, III, aVF, aVL, and V3–V6
Infarct: Pathological Q-waves in V1 and V2

This ECG demonstrates normal sinus rhythm (NSR), as the P-waves in Leads I, II, and aVF are positive, and the P-wave in Lead V1 is biphasic. The ST-segment elevations (STEs) in Leads aVR, V1, and V2, as well as small pathological Q-waves in Leads V1 and V2 represent a possible left main coronary artery (LMCA) ST-segment elevation myocardial infarction (STEMI). Similar ECG findings can be found in patients with global myocardial ischemia without LMCA plaque rupture. There are reciprocal T-wave inversions (TWIs) and ST-segment depressions (STDs) along Leads I, II, III, aVF, aVL, and V3–V6. An rSR' is present in Lead V1, and the QRS complex is >120 ms in duration, which is consistent with a right bundle branch block (RBBB).

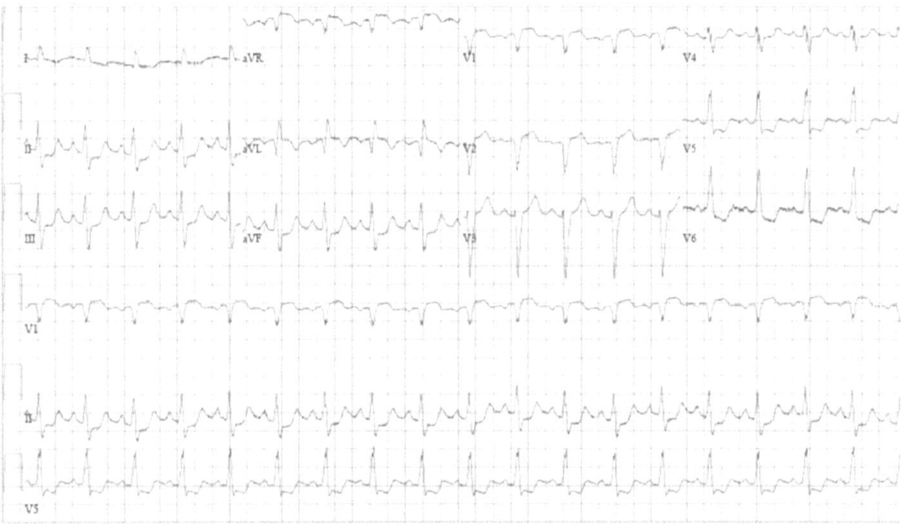

FIGURE 9.99

Rhythm: Sinus tachycardia
Rate: 117 BPM
Axis: Normal (Physiological)
Intervals: Normal
P-wave: Normal
QRS Complex: Right bundle branch block (RBBB)
T-wave: ST-segment elevations (STEs) in Leads aVR, V1, and V2, T-wave inversions (TWIs) and ST-segment depressions (STDs) in Leads I, II, III, aVF, aVL, and V4–V6
Infarct: Pathological Q-waves in V1 and V2

This ECG demonstrates normal sinus rhythm (NSR), as the P-waves in Leads I, II, and aVF are positive, and the P-wave in Lead V1 is biphasic. The ST-segment elevations (STEs) in Leads aVR, V1, and V2, as well as small pathological Q-waves in Leads V1 and V2 represent a possible left main coronary artery (LMCA) ST-segment elevation myocardial infarction (STEMI). Similar ECG findings can be found in patients with global myocardial ischemia without LMCA plaque rupture. There are reciprocal T-wave inversions (TWIs) and ST-segment depressions (STDs) along Leads I, II, III, aVF, aVL, and V4–V6. An rSR' is present in Lead V1, and the QRS complex is >120 ms in duration, which is consistent with a right bundle branch block (RBBB).

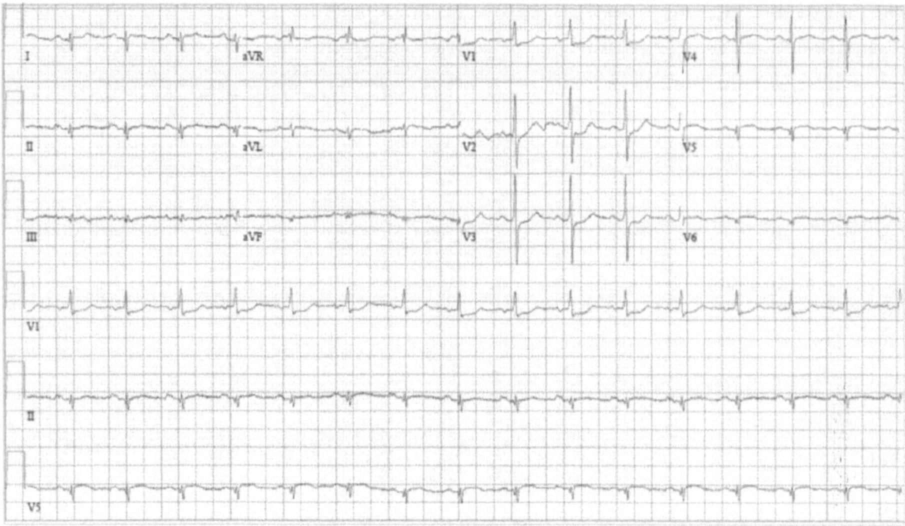

FIGURE 9.100

Rhythm: Sinus rhythm
Rate: 96 BPM
Axis: Northwestern axis deviation
Intervals: Normal
P-wave: Normal
QRS Complex: Normal
T-wave: ST-segment depressions (STDs) in Leads V1–V3
Infarct: Tall R-waves in Leads V1–V3

This ECG demonstrates normal sinus rhythm (NSR), as the P-waves in Leads I, II, and aVF are positive, and the P-wave in Lead V1 is biphasic. The R-wave amplitude is greater than the S-wave amplitude in Leads V1–V3; when there is concomitant T-wave inversion (TWI) and/or ST-segment depression (STD) on the anterior Leads in the appropriate clinical context, a posterior-wall myocardial infarction (MI) may be present. The QRS axis on this tracing is a Northwestern axis (also known as an extreme right axis, or a superior axis), due to the S-waves in both Leads I and II being greater in amplitude than their respective R-waves. Additionally, the amplitude of the QRS complex in the limb Leads does not exceed 1 large box (5 mm), which is consistent with low voltage.

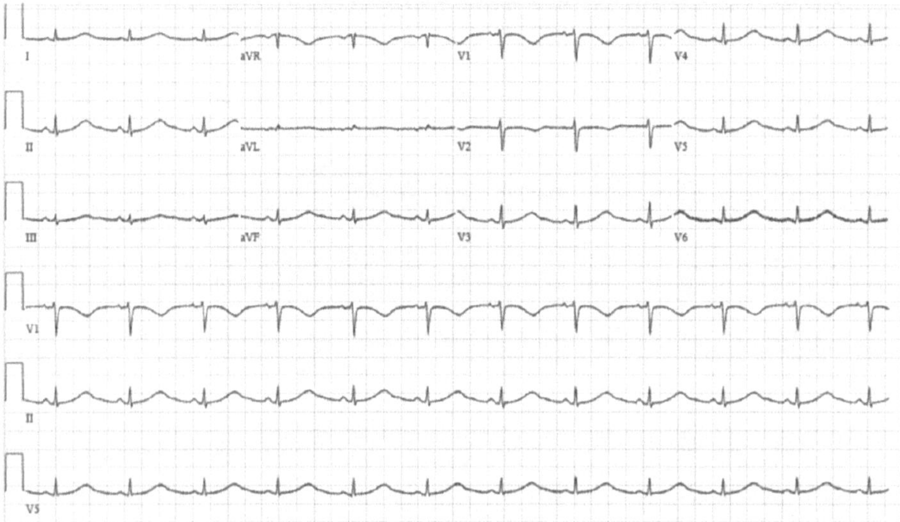

FIGURE 9.101

Rhythm: Sinus rhythm
Rate: 70 BPM
Axis: Normal (Physiologic)
Intervals: QT-interval prolongation >500 ms
P-wave: Normal
QRS Complex: Low voltage
T-wave: Normal
Infarct: None

This ECG demonstrates normal sinus rhythm (NSR), as the P-waves in Leads I, II, and aVF are positive, and the P-wave in Lead V1 is biphasic. The corrected QT-interval (QTc) is prolonged in this tracing, being >450 ms in duration. In this particular ECG, the QTc (using Bazett's formula) is in excess of 500 ms, with the uncorrected QT-interval being >550 ms. Additionally, QRS complexes <10 mm in amplitude throughout the precordial leads are consistent with low voltage. A QRS complex amplitude of 6 mm in Lead II prevents the limb leads from being labeled as low voltage (<5 mm in amplitude along the limb leads).

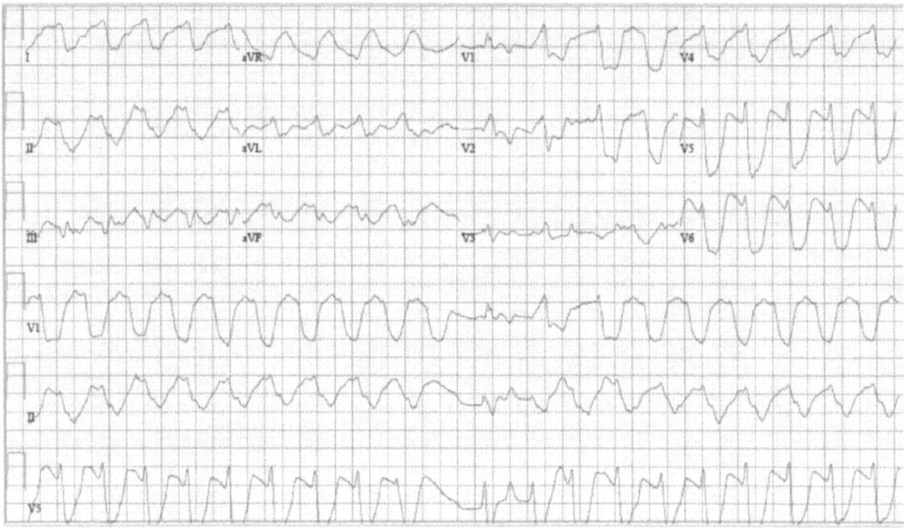

FIGURE 9.102

Rhythm: Sinusoidal rhythm
Rate: 116 BPM
Axis: Unable to assess
Intervals: Unable to assess
P-wave: Unable to assess
QRS Complex: Markedly wide QRS complex >200 ms
T-wave: Unable to assess
Infarct: None

This tracing demonstrates a sinusoidal rhythm, where most of the architecture of the tracing has been lost. Sinusoidal rhythms are indicative of underlying severe hyperkalemia, typically with serum potassium concentrations greater than 7 mEq/L.

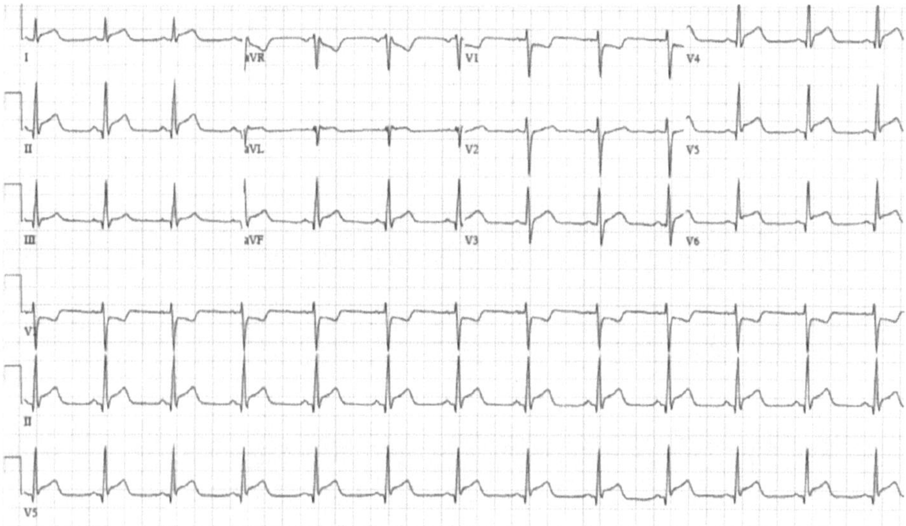

FIGURE 9.103

Rhythm: Sinus rhythm, Acute pericarditis
Rate: 76 BPM
Axis: Normal (Physiologic)
Intervals: Diffuse ST-segment elevations (STEs)
P-wave: Normal
QRS Complex: Normal
T-wave: Normal
Infarct: None

This ECG demonstrates normal sinus rhythm (NSR), as the P-waves in Leads I, II, and aVF are positive. There are diffuse ST-segment elevations present in Leads I, aVL, II, III, aVF, and V3–V6 that are all 2–3 mm in amplitude, in the absence of pathological Q-waves or reciprocal ST-segment depressions. There are no significant PR-segment depressions or PR-segment elevations in Lead aVR, which may be seen in some cases. Collectively, these ECG changes are indicative of acute pericarditis.

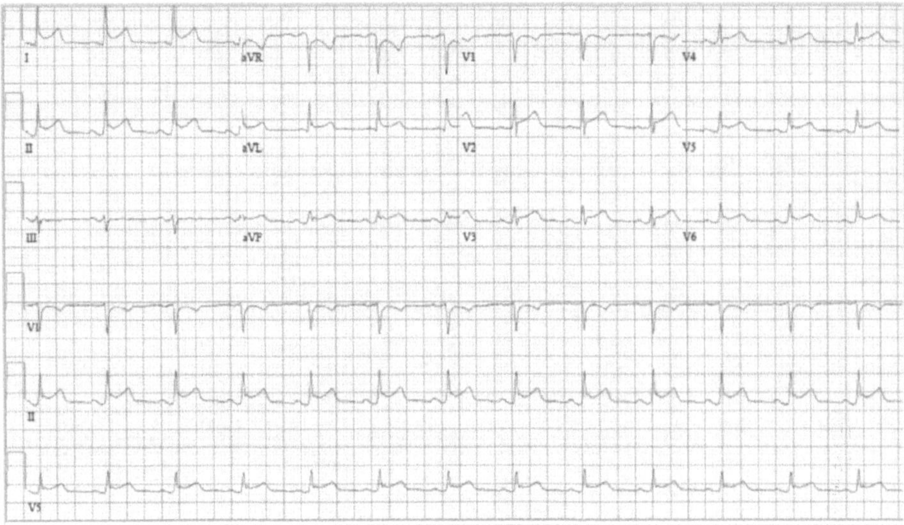

FIGURE 9.104

Rhythm: Sinus rhythm, Acute pericarditis
Rate: 78 BPM
Axis: Normal (Physiologic)
Intervals: Diffuse ST-segment Elevations (STEs)
P-wave: Normal
QRS Complex: Normal
T-wave: Normal
Infarct: None

This ECG demonstrates normal sinus rhythm (NSR), as the P-waves in Leads I, II, and aVF are positive. There are diffuse ST-segment elevations present in Leads I, aVL, II, III, aVF, and V3–V6 that are all >1 mm in amplitude, in the absence of pathological Q-waves or reciprocal ST-segment depressions (STDs). Additionally, there are diffuse PR-segment depressions as well as a PR-segment elevation in Lead aVR. Collectively, these ECG changes are indicative of acute pericarditis.

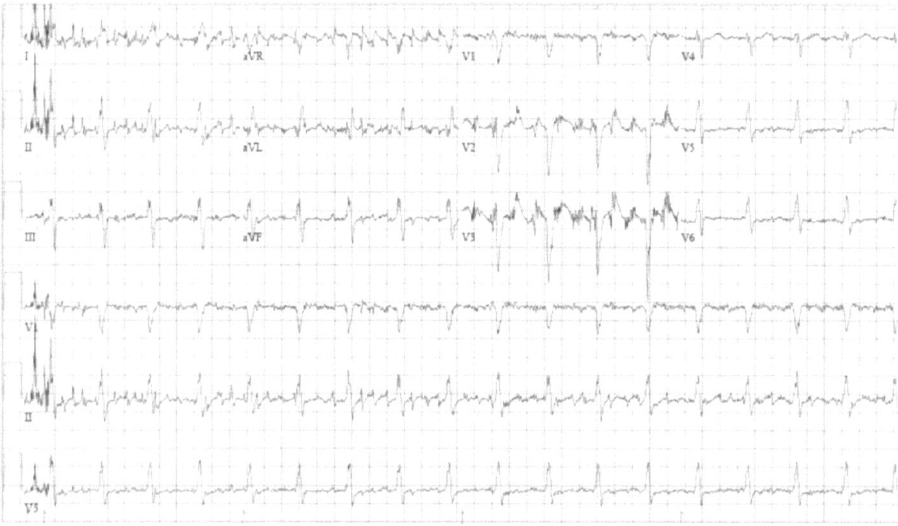

FIGURE 9.105

Rhythm: Sinus tachycardia
Rate: 108 BPM
Axis: Normal (Physiologic)
Intervals: Normal
P-wave: Normal
QRS Complex: Poor R-wave progression (PRWP), Intraventricular conduction delay (IVCD)
T-wave: Normal
Infarct: None

This ECG demonstrates normal sinus rhythm (NSR), as the P-waves in Leads I, II, and aVF are positive. The voltage spikes that are seen along the tracing represent a motion artifact from a resting tremor in this patient with Parkinson's disease. Poor R-wave progression (PRWP) is present along the precordial leads, as the QRS complex does not become positive until Lead V5, with the isoelectric point between Leads V4 and V5. There is a nonspecific intraventricular conduction delay (IVCD), which is seen with a QRS complex duration of >110 ms in the absence of full morphological criteria for a left or right bundle branch block (LBBB/RBBB).

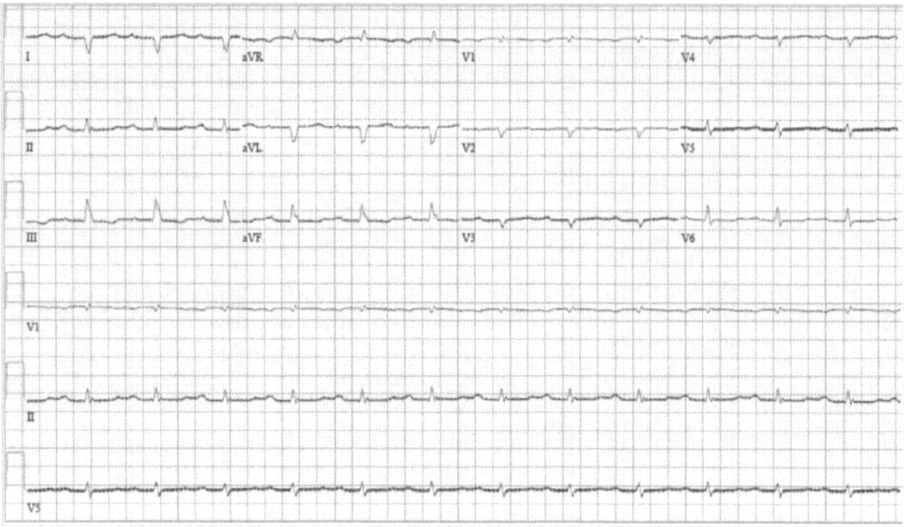

FIGURE 9.106

Rhythm: Sinus rhythm
Rate: 70 BPM
Axis: Normal (Physiologic)
Intervals: 1st Degree atrioventricular (AV) Delay, QTc prolongation >500 ms
P-wave: Normal
QRS Complex: Normal
T-wave: Normal
Infarct: None

This ECG demonstrates normal sinus rhythm (NSR), as the P-waves in Leads I, II, and aVF are positive. The PR interval is >200 ms, which is indicative of a 1st degree atrioventricular (AV) delay. Poor R-wave progression (PRWP) is present along the precordial leads, as the QRS complex does not become positive until Lead V5, with the isoelectric point between Leads V4 and V5. The corrected QT-interval (QTc) is prolonged in this tracing, being ~500 ms in duration. Additionally, QRS complexes <5 mm in amplitude throughout the limb leads and <10 mm in amplitude throughout the precordial leads are consistent with low voltage.

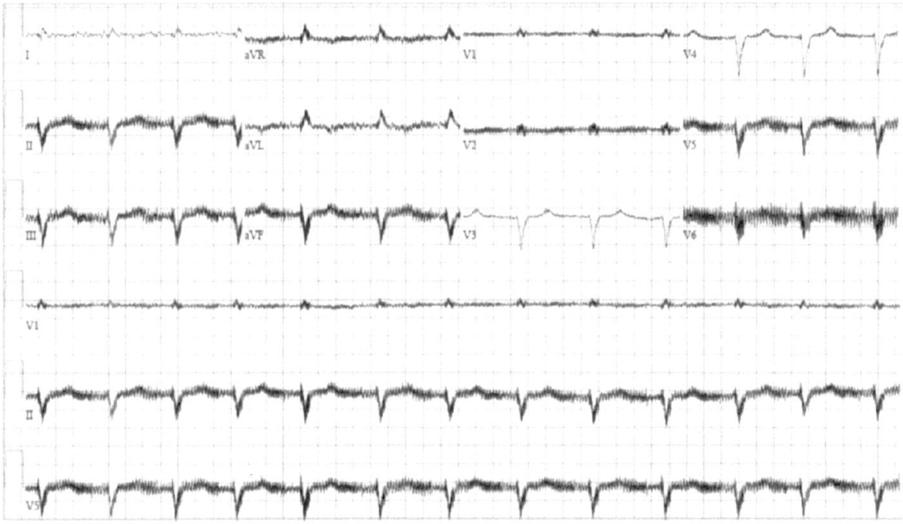

FIGURE 9.107

Rhythm: Undetermined rhythm
Rate: 75 BPM
Axis: Left axis deviation (LAD)
Intervals: Normal
P-wave: Unable to assess
QRS Complex: Poor R-wave progression (PRWP)
T-wave: Normal
Infarct: None

This rhythm of this ECG is difficult to determine, as the artifact from this patent's LVAD is obscuring the baseline. Poor R-wave progression (PRWP) is present along the precordial leads, as the QRS complex does not become positive throughout the precordium. There is a left axis deviation (LAD) present in this ECG as well, as indicated by the R-wave amplitude > S-wave amplitude in Lead I, in contrast to the R-wave amplitude < S-wave amplitude in Lead II. Finally, this patient is a recipient of a left ventricular assist device (LVAD), which explains the thickness of the lines in this tracing. The "hum" of the LVAD registers on the ECG leads, causing the above artifact.

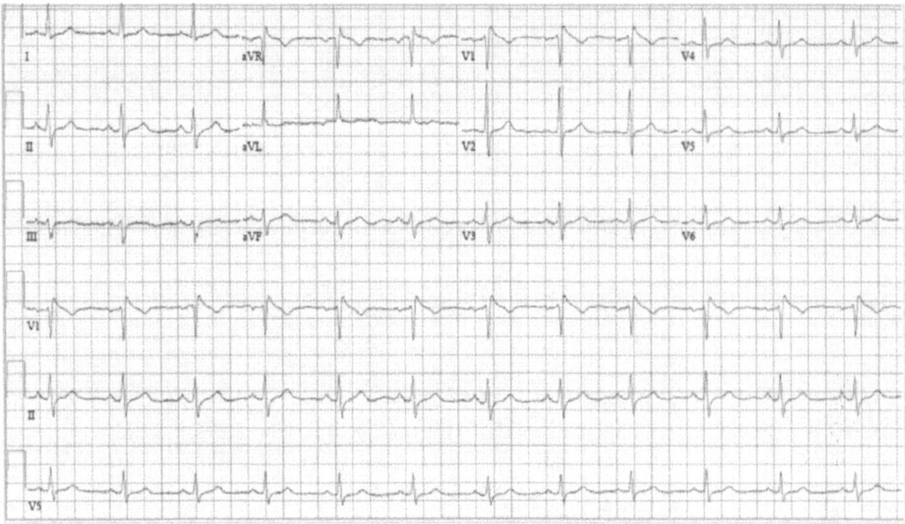

FIGURE 9.108

Rhythm: Sinus rhythm
Rate: 72 BPM
Axis: Normal (Physiological)
Intervals: Normal
P-wave: Normal
QRS Complex: Brugada syndrome, Type I pattern
T-wave: Normal
Infarct: None

This ECG demonstrates normal sinus rhythm (NSR), as the P-waves in Leads I, II, and aVF are positive. This tracing displays a Type 1 Brugada Syndrome pattern due to the "coved" ST segment and T-wave in Lead V1.

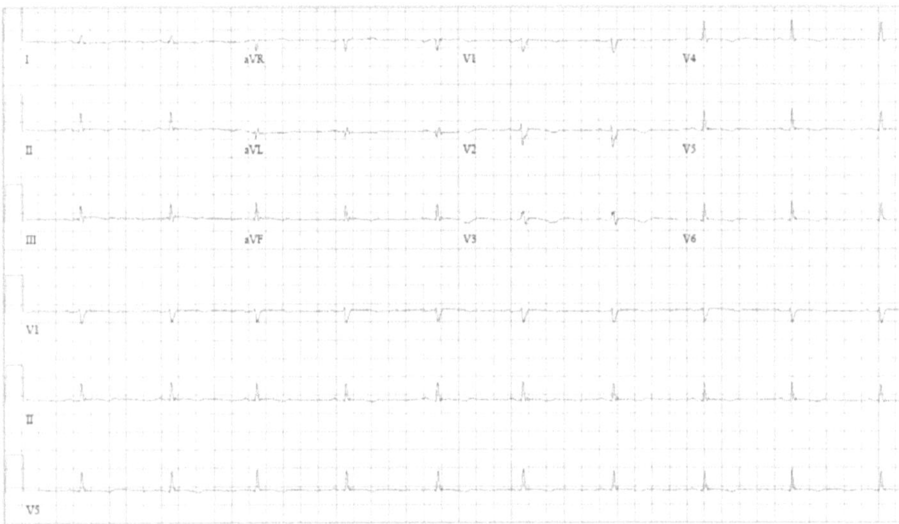

FIGURE 9.109

Rhythm: Sinus rhythm
Rate: 61 BPM
Axis: Normal (Physiological)
Intervals: Normal
P-wave: Normal
QRS Complex: Low voltage
T-wave: T-wave inversions (TWIs) in Leads V1–V6
Infarct: None

This ECG demonstrates normal sinus rhythm (NSR), as the P-waves in Leads I, II, and aVF are positive. T-wave inversions (TWIs) are present along the anterior Leads, V1–V6.

Additionally, QRS complexes <5 mm in amplitude throughout the limb leads and <10 mm in amplitude throughout the precordial leads are consistent with low voltage. Taken together, this tracing is most consistent with arrhythmogenic right ventricular cardiomyopathy (ARVC). The most specific finding of ARVC on ECG is an epsilon wave (not pictured here), which is a small, positive deflection after the QRS, best viewed in the anterior Leads.

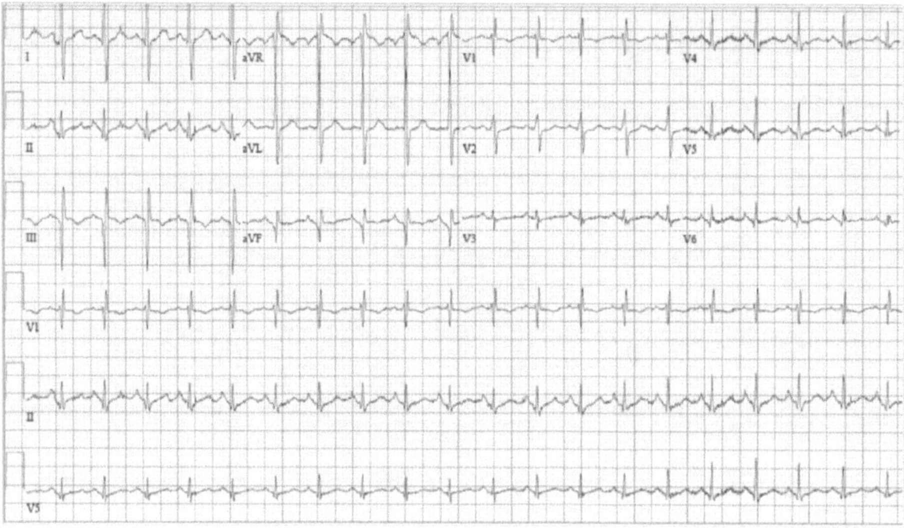

FIGURE 9.110

Rhythm: Sinus tachycardia
Rate: 120 BPM
Axis: Right axis deviation (RAD)
Intervals: Normal
P-wave: Normal
QRS Complex: Normal
T-wave: Normal
Infarct: None

This ECG demonstrates normal sinus rhythm (NSR), as the P-waves in Leads I, II, and aVF are positive. An rSR' morphology is present in Lead V1 in conjunction with a QRS complex of <120 ms in duration. This is indicative of an incomplete right bundle branch block (incomplete RBBB). Furthermore, a right axis deviation (RAD) is present, as the S-wave in Lead I is greater in amplitude than the corresponding R-wave, while the QRS complex in Lead II is positive in polarity. There is a prominent S-wave in Lead I, as well as a Q-wave and isolated T-wave inversion (TWI) in Lead III. This constellation of symptoms is known as an S1Q3T3 and is most compatible with an acute pulmonary embolism.

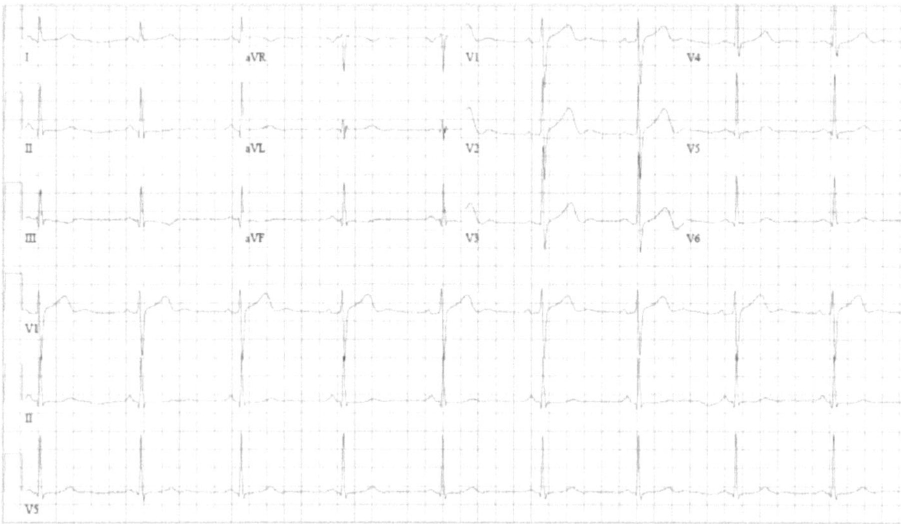

FIGURE 9.111

Rhythm: Sinus bradycardia
Rate: 55 BPM
Axis: Normal (Physiological)
Intervals: Normal
P-wave: Normal
QRS Complex: Normal
T-wave: T-wave inversions (TWIs) in Leads III and aVF, U-waves
Infarct: None

This ECG demonstrates normal sinus rhythm (NSR), as the P-waves in Leads I, II, and aVF are positive. U-waves are present embedded into the end of each T-wave (these are best appreciated in the precordial Leads). T-wave inversions (TWIs) are present in Leads III and aVF, which may represent ischemia.

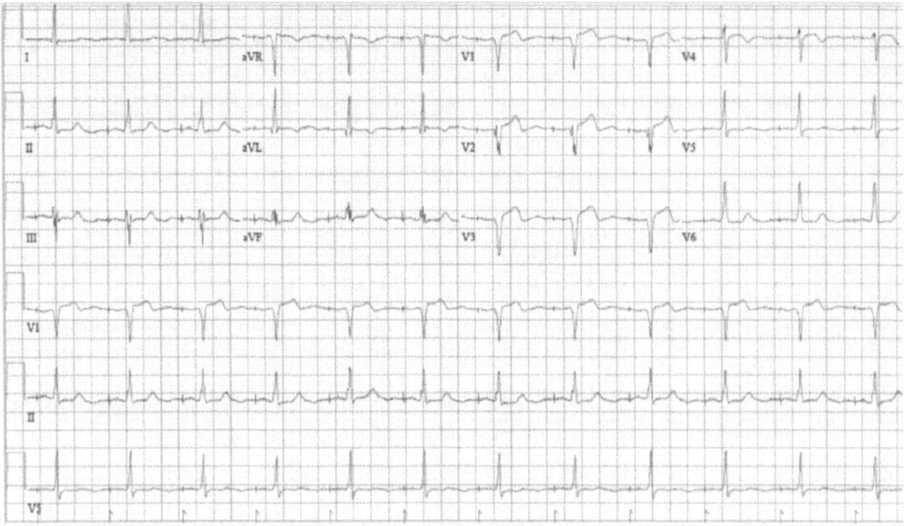

FIGURE 9.112

Rhythm: Sinus rhythm; Atrial-pacing, Permanent pacemaker
Rate: 72 BPM
Axis: Normal (Physiological)
Intervals: ST-segment elevations (STEs) in Leads V1–V3
P-wave: Normal
QRS Complex: Poor R-wave progression (PRWP)
T-wave: None
Infarct: Pathological Q-waves in Leads V1–V3

This ECG demonstrates a single chamber pacemaker that is atrial-pacing. This is apparent from the presence of sinus P-waves that have antecedent pacemaker spikes. As a result, this tracing represents normal sinus rhythm (NSR), as the P-waves in Leads I, II, and aVF are positive. There are pathological Q-waves in Leads V1–V3 with associated ST-segment elevations (STEs). These findings are most consistent with an anteroseptal myocardial infarction (MI) with a residual left ventricular (LV) aneurysm.

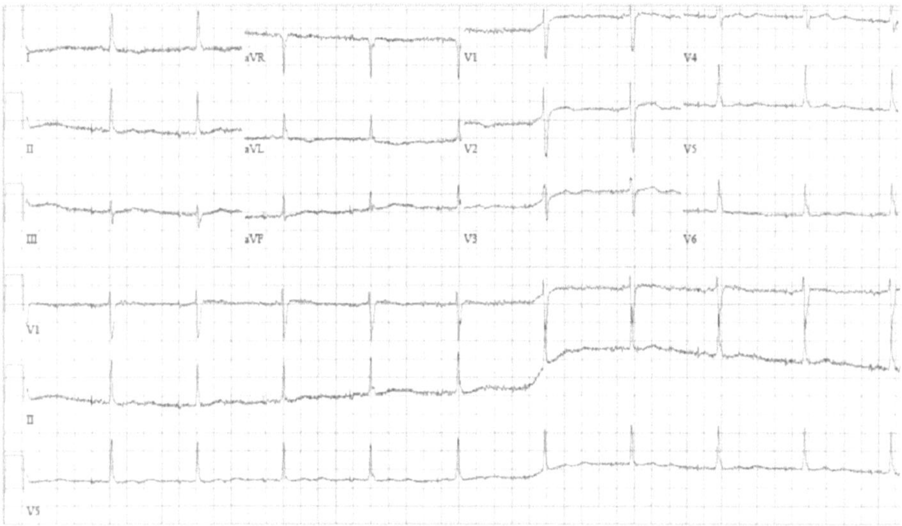

FIGURE 9.113

Rhythm: Sinus rhythm; Atrial-pacing, Permanent pacemaker
Rate: 60 BPM
Axis: Normal (Physiological)
Intervals: Normal
P-wave: Normal
QRS Complex: Normal
T-wave: Diffuse Nonspecific T-wave flattening
Infarct: None

This ECG demonstrates a single chamber pacemaker that is atrial-pacing. This is apparent from the presence of sinus P-waves that have antecedent pacemaker spikes. As a result, this tracing represents normal sinus rhythm (NSR), as the P-waves in Leads I, II, and aVF are positive. There are diffuse, nonspecific T-wave inversions (TWIs).

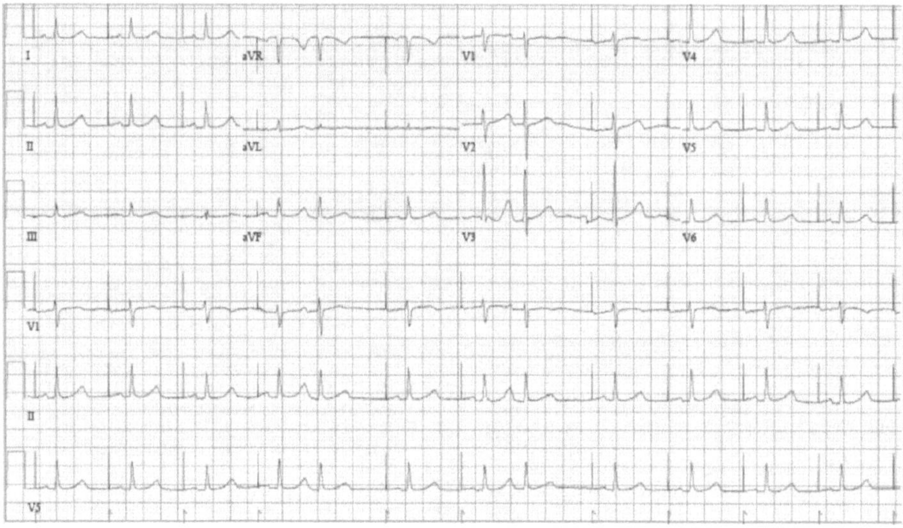

FIGURE 9.114

Rhythm: Sinus rhythm; Atrial-sensing and pacing, Permanent pacemaker
Rate: 60 BPM
Axis: Normal (Physiological)
Intervals: Normal
P-wave: Normal
QRS Complex: Poor R-Wave progression (PRWP)
T-wave: None
Infarct: None

This ECG demonstrates a single chamber pacemaker that is atrial-sensing and pacing. This is apparent from the presence of sinus P-waves that have antecedent pacemaker spikes. However, the lack of pacing spikes prior to the premature atrial contractions (PACs) that represent the 5th and 8th beats on the rhythm strips implies that the device is also atrial-sensing. This tracing represents normal sinus rhythm (NSR), as the P-waves in Leads I, II, and aVF are positive.

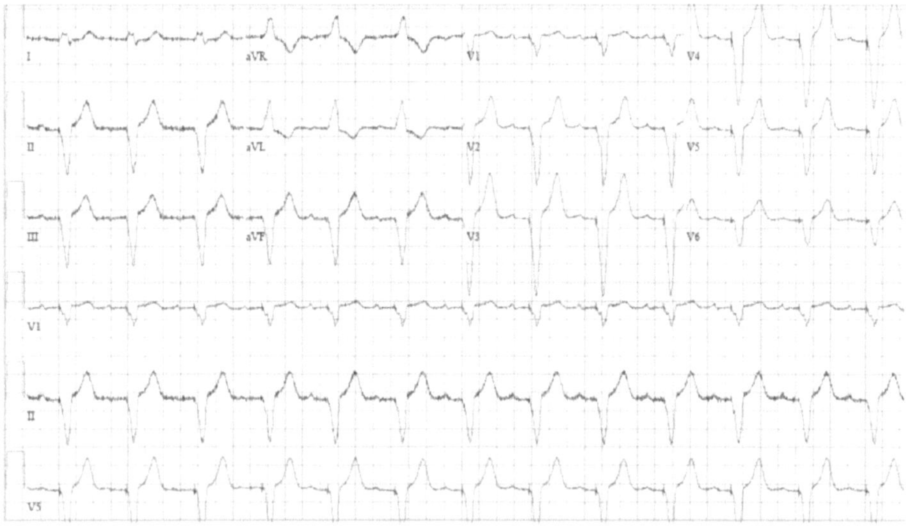

FIGURE 9.115

Rhythm: Sinus rhythm; Ventricular pacing, Permanent pacemaker
Rate: 60 BPM
Axis: Left axis deviation (LAD)
Intervals: 1st Degree atrioventricular (AV) delay
P-wave: Normal
QRS Complex: Ventricular pacing
T-wave: None
Infarct: None

This ECG likely demonstrates a dual-chamber pacemaker that is ventricular-pacing. This is apparent from the presence of left bundle branch morphology QRS complexes that have antecedent pacemaker spikes. The left bundle branch morphology is evidence that this pacemaker is dual-chambered. This tracing represents normal sinus rhythm (NSR), as the P-waves in Leads I, II, and aVF are positive. The PR interval is >200 ms, which is indicative of a 1st degree atrioventricular (AV) delay. There is a left axis deviation (LAD) present in this ECG as well, as indicated by the R-wave amplitude > S-wave amplitude in Lead I, in contrast to the R-wave amplitude < S-wave amplitude in Lead II.

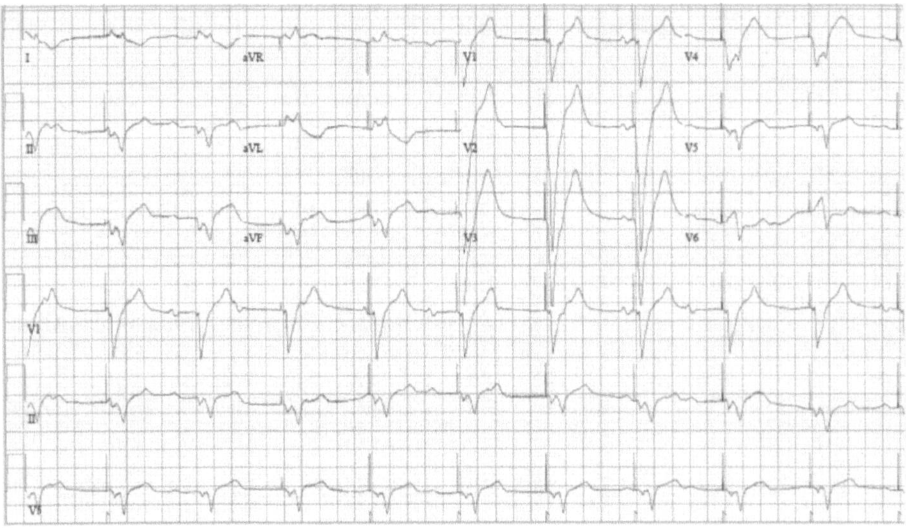

FIGURE 9.116

Rhythm: Sinus rhythm; Ventricular pacing, Temporary venous pacing (TVP) wire
Rate: 60 BPM
Axis: Left axis deviation (LAD)
Intervals: Constant PP and RR intervals
P-wave: Normal
QRS Complex: Ventricular pacing
T-wave: None
Infarct: None

This ECG demonstrates a temporary venous pacing wire that is ventricular-sensing and pacing. This is apparent from the presence of left bundle branch morphology QRS complexes that have antecedent pacemaker spikes. However, the lack of an antecedent pacemaker spike prior to the 3rd beat in the tracing implies that the device is also ventricular sensing. This tracing represents normal sinus rhythm (NSR), as the P-waves in Leads I, II, and aVF are positive. There are P-waves throughout the rhythm strip that do not conduct to an associated QRS complex. However, the PP-interval and RR-interval remain constant throughout the tracing, while the PR-interval varies. The atrial rate (around 80 BPM) is faster than the ventricular rate (paced around 60 BPM); the atria and the ventricles are depolarizing independently of one another. This pattern of AV dissociation in the context of an atrial rate faster than the ventricular rate is consistent with 3rd degree atrioventricular block (AVB), otherwise known as complete heart block (CHB). There is a left axis deviation (LAD) present in this ECG as well, as indicated by the R-wave amplitude > S-wave amplitude in Lead I, in contrast to the R-wave amplitude < S-wave amplitude in Lead II.

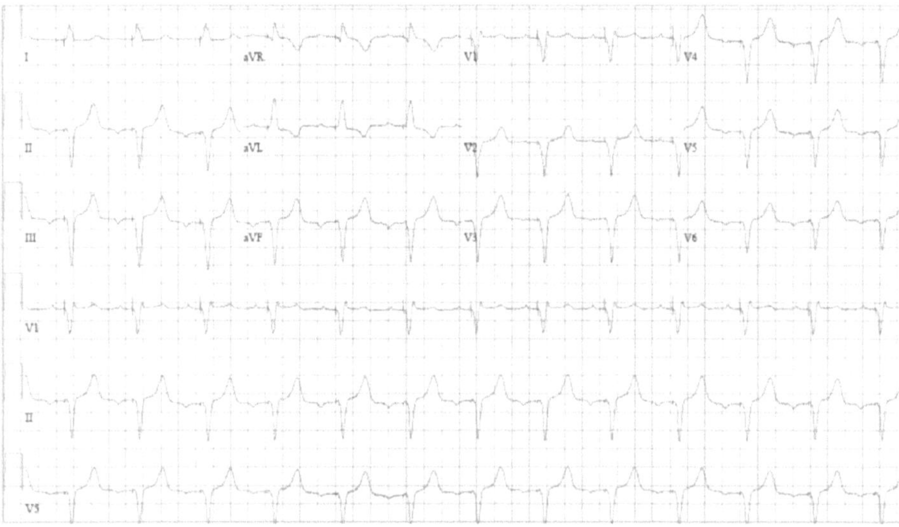

FIGURE 9.117

Rhythm: Ectopic atrial rhythm; Ventricular pacing, Permanent pacemaker
Rate: 77 BPM
Axis: Left axis deviation (LAD)
Intervals: 1st Degree atrioventricular (AV) delay
P-wave: Ectopic
QRS Complex: Ventricular pacing
T-wave: None
Infarct: None

This ECG likely demonstrates a dual chamber pacemaker that is ventricular-pacing. This is apparent from the presence of left bundle branch morphology QRS complexes that have antecedent pacemaker spikes. Additionally, this tracing has a regular RR interval but is not indicative of sinus rhythm. The P-waves within Leads II, III, and aVF are inverted (negative amplitude) and, as such, cannot be originating from the sinoatrial (SA) node. This pattern is most consistent with an ectopic atrial rhythm. The PR interval is >200 ms, which is indicative of a 1st degree atrioventricular (AV) delay. There is a left axis deviation (LAD) present in this ECG as well, as indicated by the R-wave amplitude > S-wave amplitude in Lead I, in contrast to the R-wave amplitude < S-wave amplitude in Lead II.

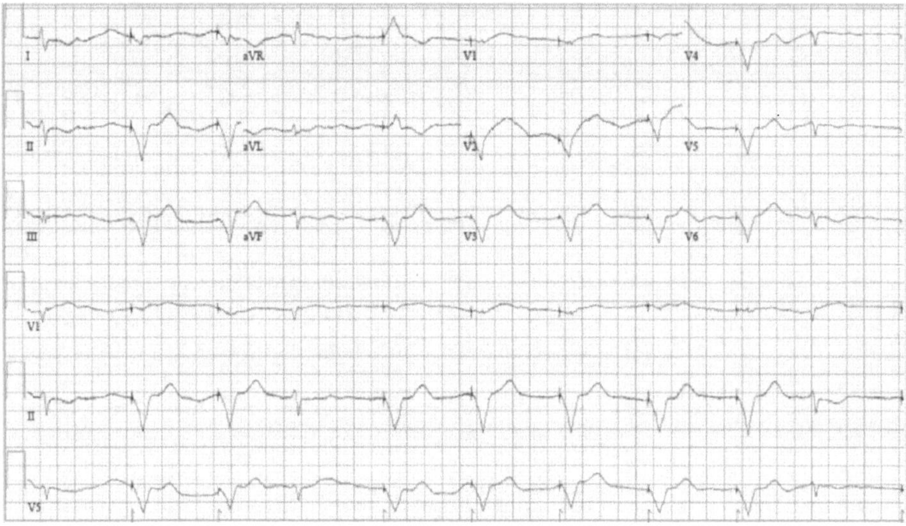

FIGURE 9.118

Rhythm: Atrial fibrillation with a controlled ventricular response (CVR); Ventricular pacing, Permanent pacemaker
Rate: 65 BPM
Axis: Northwestern axis deviation
Intervals: Normal
P-wave: Not applicable
QRS Complex: Ventricular pacing
T-wave: T-wave inversions (TWIs) in Leads V4–V6
Infarct: None

This ECG likely demonstrates a dual-chamber pacemaker that is ventricular-pacing. This is apparent from the presence of left bundle branch morphology QRS complexes that have antecedent pacemaker spikes. The left bundle branch morphology is evidence that this pacemaker is dual-chambered. However, the lack of an antecedent pacemaker spike prior to the 1st, 4th, and 10th beats in the tracing implies that the device is also ventricular sensing. This ECG demonstrates a lack of discernable P-waves amidst a random oscillation of electrical activity along the baseline, which is consistent with atrial fibrillation (Afib). The f-waves (fibrillatory waves) are characterized by random deflections that vary in terms of duration, amplitude, and morphology. This is associated with an irregularly irregular RR interval with a controlled ventricular response (CVR), due to the ventricular heart rate between 60 BPM and 100 BPM. The QRS axis on this tracing is a Northwestern axis (also known as an extreme right axis, or a superior axis), due to the S-waves in both Leads I and II being greater in amplitude than their respective R-waves. When unpaced, there are T-wave inversions (TWIs) in Leads V4–V6, possibly consistent with ischemia.

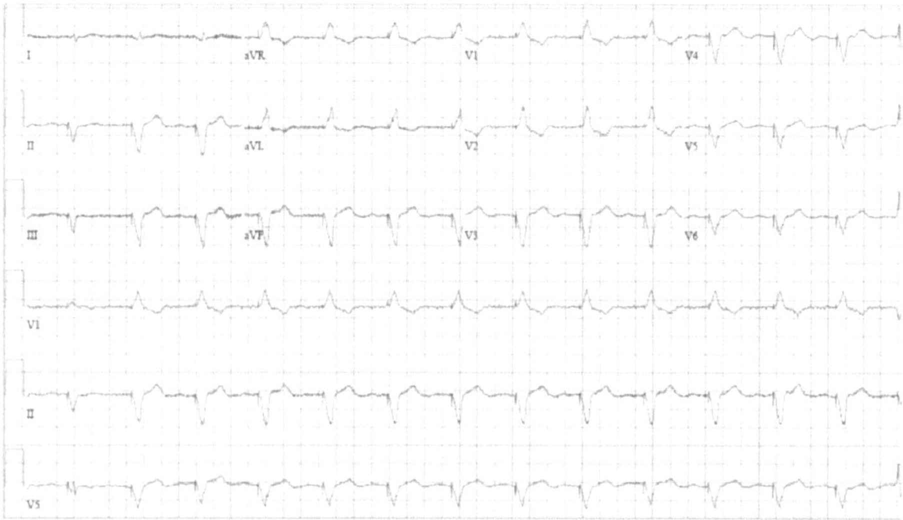

FIGURE 9.119

Rhythm: Atrial fibrillation with a controlled ventricular response (CVR); Biventricular pacing, Permanent pacemaker
Rate: 83 BPM
Axis: Left axis deviation (LAD)
Intervals: Normal
P-wave: Not applicable
QRS Complex: Biventricular pacing
T-wave: None
Infarct: None

This ECG demonstrates a biventricular pacemaker that is ventricular-pacing. This is apparent from the presence of right bundle branch morphology QRS complexes that have antecedent pacemaker spikes. The right bundle branch morphology is evidence that this pacemaker is a biventricular device. This ECG demonstrates a lack of discernable P-waves amidst a random oscillation of electrical activity along the baseline, which is consistent with atrial fibrillation (Afib). The f-waves (fibrillatory waves) are characterized by random deflections that vary in terms of duration, amplitude, and morphology. This is associated with a controlled ventricular response (CVR), due to the ventricular heart rate between 60 BPM and 100 BPM. There is a left axis deviation (LAD) present in this ECG as well, as indicated by the R-wave amplitude > S-wave amplitude in Lead I, in contrast to the R-wave amplitude < S-wave amplitude in Lead II.

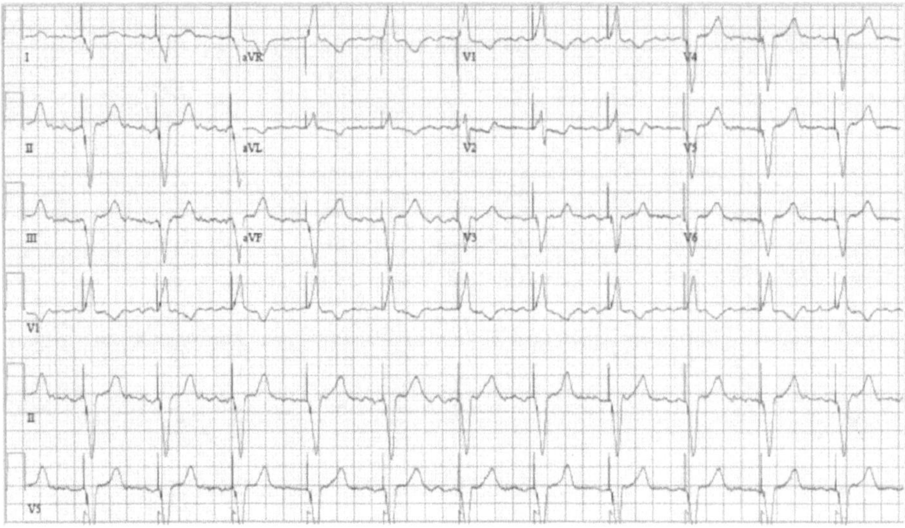

FIGURE 9.120

Rhythm: Atrial fibrillation with a controlled ventricular response (CVR); Biventricular pacing, Permanent pacemaker
Rate: 66 BPM
Axis: Northwestern axis deviation
Intervals: Normal
P-wave: Not applicable
QRS Complex: Biventricular pacing
T-wave: None
Infarct: None

This ECG demonstrates a biventricular pacemaker that is ventricular-pacing. This is apparent from the presence of right bundle branch morphology QRS complexes that have antecedent pacemaker spikes. The right bundle branch morphology is evidence that this pacemaker is a biventricular device. This ECG demonstrates a lack of discernable P-waves amidst a random oscillation of electrical activity along the baseline, which is consistent with atrial fibrillation (Afib). The f-waves (fibrillatory waves) are characterized by random deflections that vary in terms of duration, amplitude, and morphology. This is associated with a controlled ventricular response (CVR), due to the ventricular heart rate between 60 BPM and 100 BPM. The QRS axis on this tracing is a Northwestern axis (also known as an extreme right axis, or a superior axis), due to the S-waves in both Leads I and II being greater in amplitude than their respective R-waves.

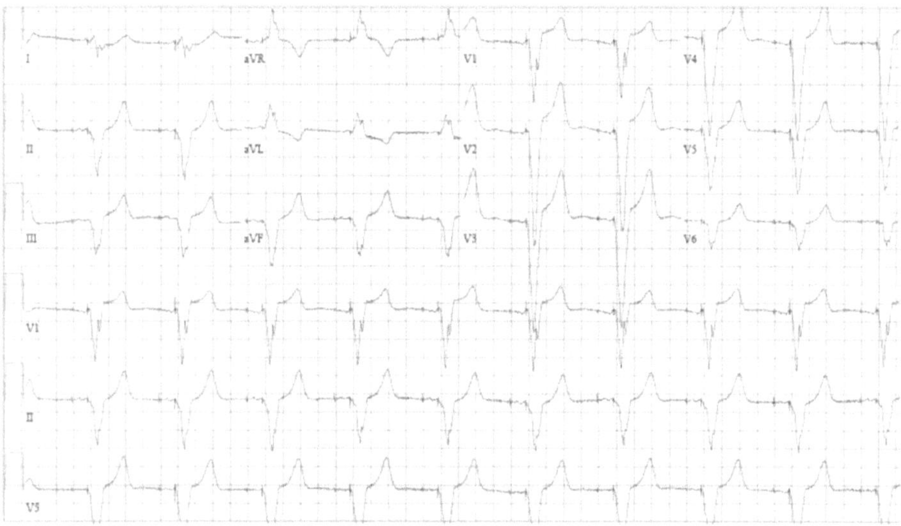

FIGURE 9.121

Rhythm: Sinus rhythm; Atrioventricular pacing, Permanent pacemaker
Rate: 60 BPM
Axis: Northwestern axis deviation
Intervals: Normal
P-wave: Normal
QRS Complex: Ventricular pacing
T-wave: None
Infarct: None

This ECG demonstrates a dual-chamber pacemaker that is atrial-ventricular sequential pacing. This is apparent from the presence of sinus P-waves that have antecedent pacemaker spikes, as well as the presence of left bundle branch morphology QRS complexes that also have antecedent pacemaker spikes. The left bundle branch morphology is evidence that this pacemaker is dual-chambered. This tracing represents normal sinus rhythm (NSR), as the P-waves in Leads I, II, and aVF are positive. The QRS axis on this tracing is a Northwestern axis (also known as an extreme right axis, or a superior axis), due to the S-waves in both Leads I and II being greater in amplitude than their respective R-waves.

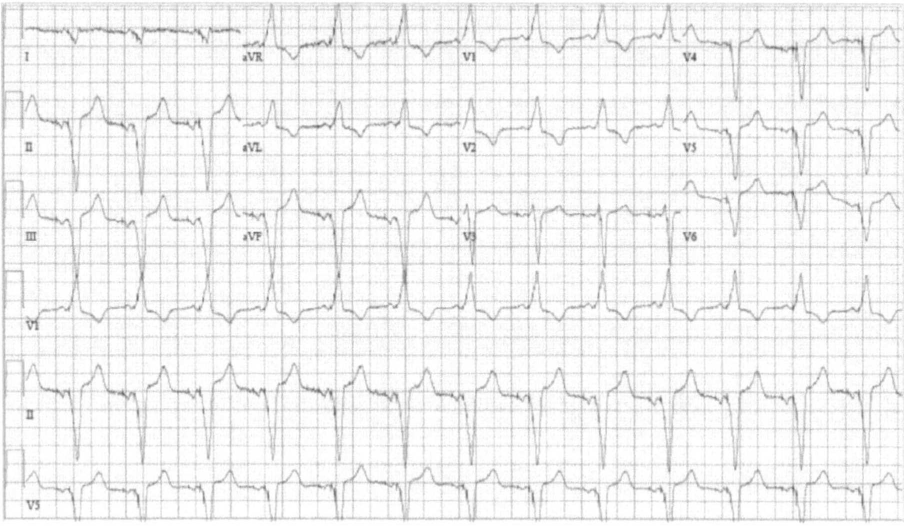

FIGURE 9.122

Rhythm: Ectopic atrial rhythm; Atrial pacing; Biventricular pacing; Permanent pacemaker
Rate: 60 BPM
Axis: Northwestern axis deviation
Intervals: Normal
P-wave: Ectopic
QRS Complex: Ventricular pacing
T-wave: None
Infarct: None

This ECG demonstrates a dual-chamber pacemaker that is atrial-ventricular sequential pacing. This is apparent from the presence of P-waves that have antecedent pacemaker spikes, as well as the presence of right bundle branch morphology QRS complexes that also have antecedent pacemaker spikes. The right bundle branch morphology is evidence that this pacemaker is a biventricular device. Additionally, this tracing has a regular RR interval but is not indicative of sinus rhythm. The P-waves within Leads II, III, and aVF are inverted (negative amplitude) and, as such, cannot be originating from the sinoatrial (SA) node. This pattern is most consistent with an ectopic atrial rhythm. The QRS axis on this tracing is a Northwestern axis (also known as an extreme right axis, or a superior axis), due to the S-waves in both Leads I and II being greater in amplitude than their respective R-waves.

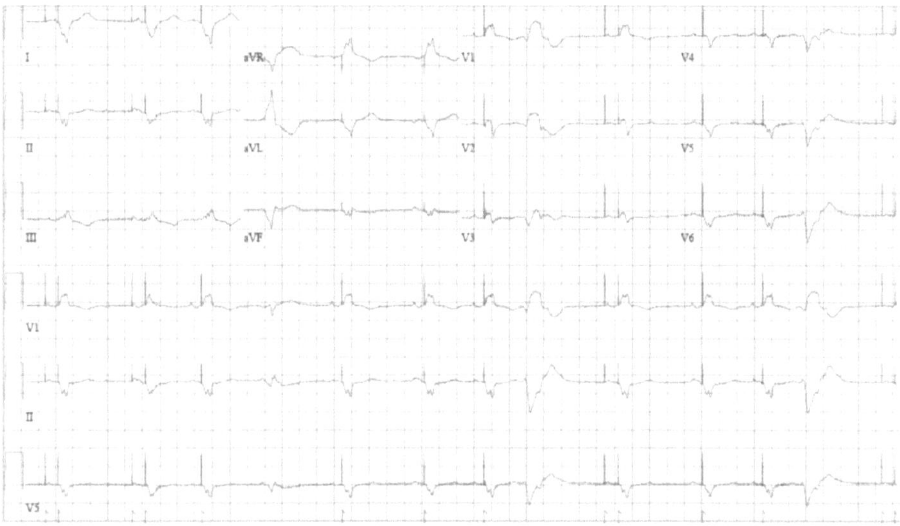

FIGURE 9.123

Rhythm: Ectopic atrial rhythm; Atrial pacing; Biventricular pacing; Permanent pacemaker
Rate: 60 BPM
Axis: Northwestern axis deviation
Intervals: Normal
P-wave: Ectopic
QRS Complex: Ventricular pacing
T-wave: None
Infarct: None

This ECG demonstrates a dual-chamber pacemaker that is atrial-ventricular sequential pacing. This is apparent from the presence of P-waves that have antecedent pacemaker spikes, as well as the presence of right bundle branch morphology QRS complexes that also have antecedent pacemaker spikes. The right bundle branch morphology is evidence that this pacemaker is a biventricular device. Additionally, this tracing has a regular RR interval but is not indicative of sinus rhythm. The P-waves within Leads II, III, and aVF are inverted (negative amplitude) and, as such, cannot be originating from the sinoatrial (SA) node. This pattern is most consistent with an ectopic atrial rhythm. The QRS axis on this tracing is a Northwestern axis (also known as an extreme right axis, or a superior axis), due to the S-waves in both Leads I and II being greater in amplitude than their respective R-waves.

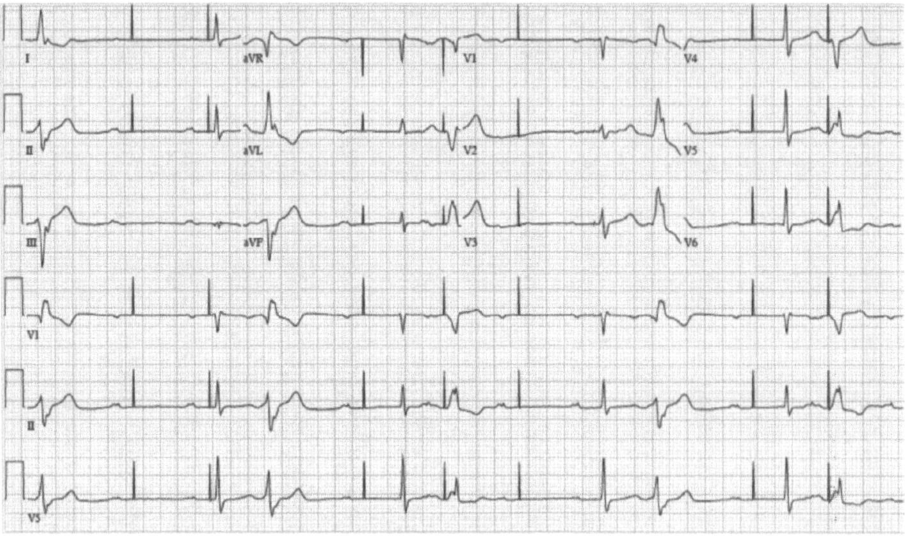

FIGURE 9.124

Rhythm: Sinus rhythm; Atrial-sensing, Ventricular-pacing, Permanent pacemaker; Failure to capture
Rate: 62 BPM
Axis: Normal (Physiologic)
Intervals: PR interval >200 ms (1st Degree AV delay)
P-wave: Left atrial abnormality (LAA)
QRS Complex: Normal, Paced
T-wave: Repolarization abnormalities from Pacemaker
Infarct: None

This ECG demonstrates a dual-chamber pacemaker that is atrial-sensing and ventricular-pacing. This is apparent from the presence of sinus P-waves that lack antecedent pacemaker "spikes." Aside from occasional conducted beats (i.e., A-sensing, V-sensing), many of the QRS complexes are preceded by pacing spikes, which is consistent with intermittent ventricular pacing. There are several ventricular pacing spikes that "fire" at the correct point in the cardiac cycle but are not associated with a QRS complex (ventricular depolarization), which is indicative of failure to capture. Occasional premature ventricular contractions (PVCs) are present, along with a prolonged PR-interval >200 ms in native beats, which is consistent with a 1st degree AV delay. The P-wave duration is borderline at ~120 ms, and the P-wave in Lead II demonstrates "notching (P-mitrale)," suggesting a left atrial abnormality (LAA) is present.

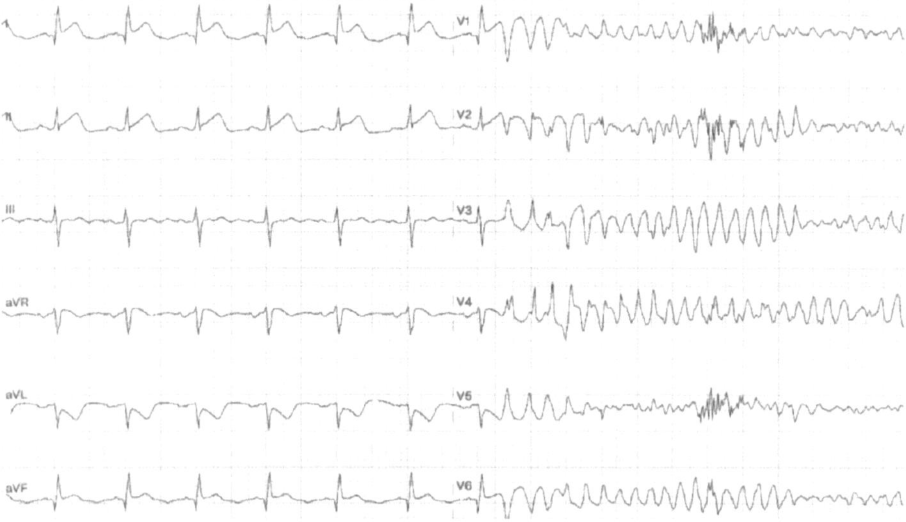

FIGURE 9.125

Rhythm: Sinus rhythm, Torsades de Pointes
Rate: 72 BPM, then >250 BPM
Axis: Normal (Physiologic)
Intervals: QT-prolongation >450 ms
P-wave: Normal
QRS Complex: Normal
T-wave: ST-segment elevations (STEs) in Leads I, II, and aVF, V1, and V2; T-wave inversions (TWIs) and ST-segment depressions (STDs) in Lead aVL
Infarct: Pathological Q-waves in Leads I, aVF, and V1

This ECG initially demonstrates normal sinus rhythm (NSR), as the P-waves in Leads I, II, and aVF are positive. The ST-segment elevations (STEs) and pathological Q-waves in Leads I, aVF, and V1 represent an evolving, acute anterolateral ST-segment elevation myocardial infarction (STEMI). There are reciprocal T-wave inversions (TWIs) and ST-segment depressions (STDs) in Lead aVL. The 8th beat in the tracing is consistent with a premature ventricular contraction (PVC) that depolarizes during the latter half of the T-wave, which corresponds to the vulnerable refractory period. This occurs on a background of borderline QTc-interval prolongation, with the corrected QTc being >450 ms. This subsequently triggers a polymorphic ventricular tachycardia (PMVT) associated with a "twisting" of the tracing, referred to as torsades de pointes.

BIBLIOGRAPHY

1. O'Keefe, J. H., Pogwizd, S. M., Freed, M. S., & Hammill, S. C. (2015). *The ECG Criteria Book* (2nd ed.). Jones & Bartlett Learning.

Question Bank* 10

Ryan F. Heslin, On Chen, and Abhijeet Singh

QUESTION BANK

Question 1

A 77-year-old Caucasian female presents to the emergency department for total loss of consciousness. She states that this is her second episode in 3 months, both without prodrome. This episode occurred 2 hours prior to presentation and was witnessed by her friend, who denies any seizure-like activity or post-ictal confusion. She states to have fully lost consciousness and estimates a downtime of approximately 10 seconds. Her prior medical history includes pre-diabetes, pre-hypertension, and depression, and she does not take any medications. Her vitals upon presentation were all within normal limits. Orthostatic vital signs were negative. Her physical exam is benign, with a normal cardiac exam, and her lab work is unremarkable. Her current ECG obtained on presentation is shown below; her baseline ECG from last year was completely normal.

* A special thank you to Ryan Heslin and Abhijeet Singh for their tireless efforts in ensuring the clinical questions in this chapter are meticulously crafted

DOI: 10.1201/9781003565383-10

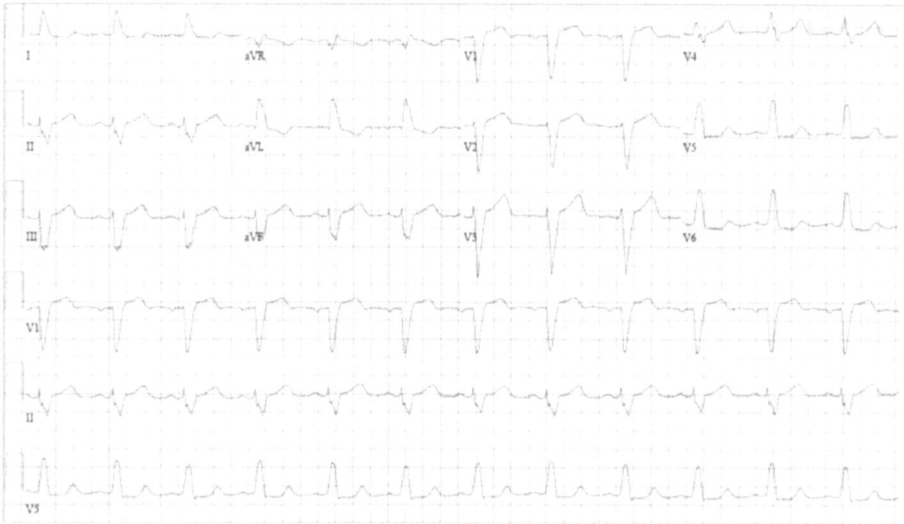

FIGURE 10.1

What does this ECG show, and what is the next best step in management?

A. NSR with RBBB; Place on a Holter monitor and outpatient recommend cardiology follow-up
B. NSR with LBBB; Reassurance and discharge given likely benign syncope
C. NSR with LBBB; Consultation with the EP service for PPM implantation
D. NSR with RBBB; Physical therapy evaluation for deconditioning
E. NSR with Bifascicular block; Electroencephalogram to rule out seizure activity

Question 2

A 46-year-old Caucasian male presents to the emergency department for chest pain. The patient states this is his second episode in the last few days. He initially noticed the pain when he was playing indoor hockey. He states he may have sustained some minor chest trauma during the game. He describes the pain was substernal in location and dull in quality without any radiation; it resolved during halftime. He woke up today and again experienced a similar pain, but now the pain is not going away. He hasn't found any relief with position or ibuprofen. The patient has a prior medical history of dyslipidemia, anxiety, and former tobacco use disorder. He is not on any long-term prescription medications. His vitals are stable. His physical exam is significant for distress secondary to pain and xanthelasmas on his eyelids. The nursing assistant hands you the ECG pictured below.

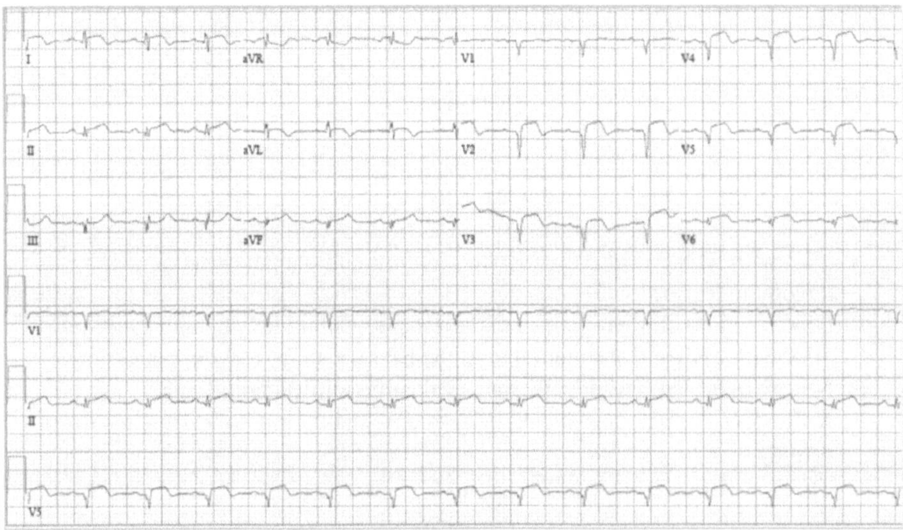

FIGURE 10.2

What does the ECG show, and what is the next appropriate step in the management of this patient?

A. Artifact; Ask the nursing assistant to repeat the ECG to obtain a better tracing
B. STEMI; Initiate STEMI protocol and load the patient with aspirin
C. STEMI; Order for an echocardiogram for evaluation of a pericardial effusion
D. Pericarditis; Start the patient on NSAIDs for likely pericarditis
E. Pericarditis; Obtain a chest XR in multiple views for evaluation of rib fractures

Question 3

A 64-year-old Caucasian female presents to the primary care clinic for management of her chronic medical problems. She has no complaints and is adherent to her medications. She has a past medical history of hypertension, hypothyroidism, and sleep apnea. Her vitals today are significant for a blood pressure of 148/83, and her cardiac exam reveals a regular rate and rhythm, without murmurs, rubs, or gallops. You obtain an ECG as part of her annual visit, which is shown below. The patient asks if she is at risk for any "heart problems" based on her ECG.

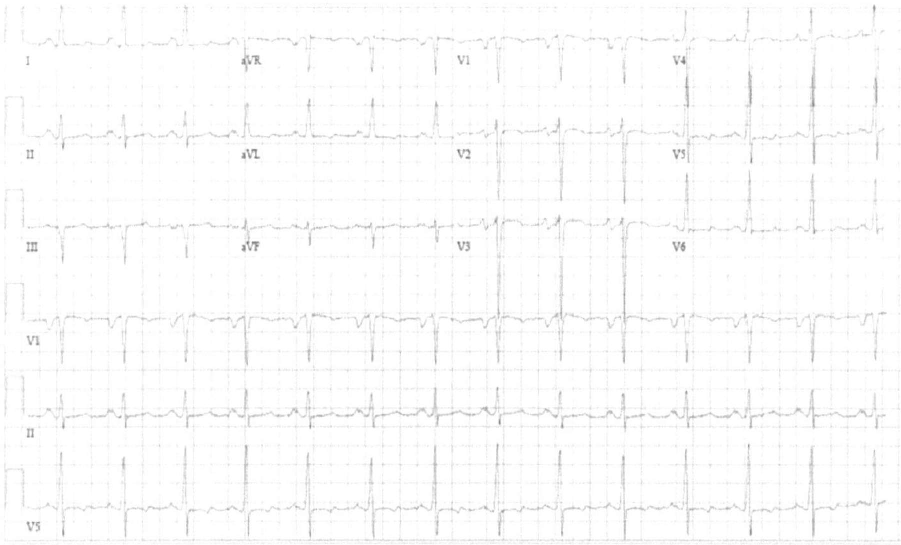

FIGURE 10.3

What does the ECG show, and what condition is this finding associated with?

A. Left atrial enlargement; Atrial fibrillation
B. Low voltage QRS; Congestive heart failure
C. Right bundle branch block; Pulmonary hypertension
D. T-wave inversions; Myocardial infarction
E. No abnormalities; Her ECG looks perfect

Question 4

A 62-year-old Caucasian male presents to the primary care clinic for follow-up. Approximately 1 week ago, he started noticing a productive cough with subjective fevers. After going to the urgent care clinic, he was started on azithromycin and steroids 2 days ago for a presumed URI. Today he feels better, with improvement in his cough and sputum production. He has a medical history of hypertension, chronic obstructive pulmonary disease, and multiple mood disorders. He takes his medications regularly and requests refills for his haloperidol and sertraline. His vitals are stable, and he is afebrile. Examination of his lungs is without any rales, rhonchi, or egophony. His ECG is shown below.

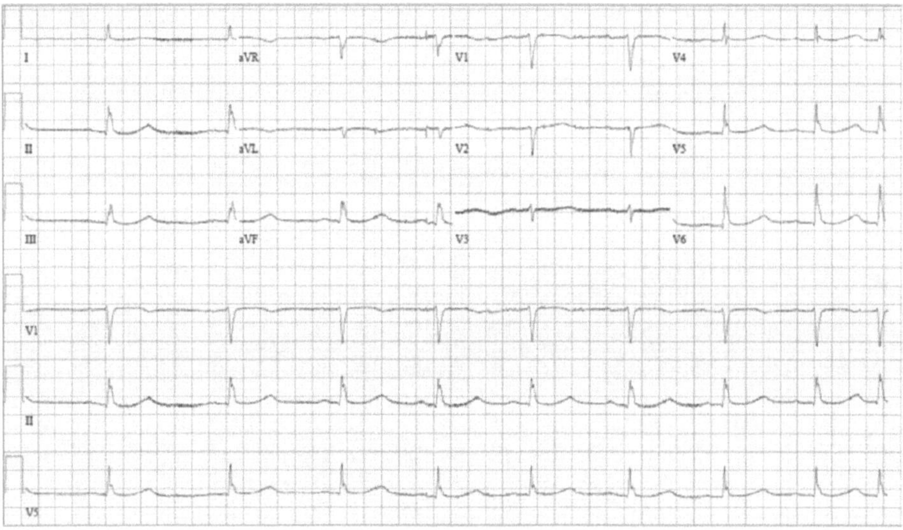

FIGURE 10.4

What does the ECG show, and what is the best next step in management?

A. QT Prolongation; Ask to see the patient in 6 months for routine follow-up and the influenza vaccination
B. NSR with LVH; Tell the patient to continue the azithromycin and present to the nearest ED for evaluation
C. QT Prolongation; Discontinue the azithromycin and re-evaluate his medication regimen
D. LBBB; Order a Holter monitor for 30 days to evaluate for additional conduction abnormalities
E. Torsades de Pointes; Tell the patient to stop his SSRI and haloperidol and re-evaluate his medication regimen

Question 5

An 80-year-old male presents to the emergency department for evaluation of intermittent lightheadedness. He has a medical history of atrial fibrillation status post-pacemaker implantation and recent diagnosis of an acute deep vein thrombosis on apixaban. The patient states that for the last several days he has been feeling lightheaded but denies any falls or loss of consciousness. His vitals are stable, and his physical exam is significant for a normal cardiac exam and negative orthostatic vital signs. His lab work is without any abnormalities. His CXR shows a pacemaker in the left hemithorax but without any acute findings. His ECG is shown below.

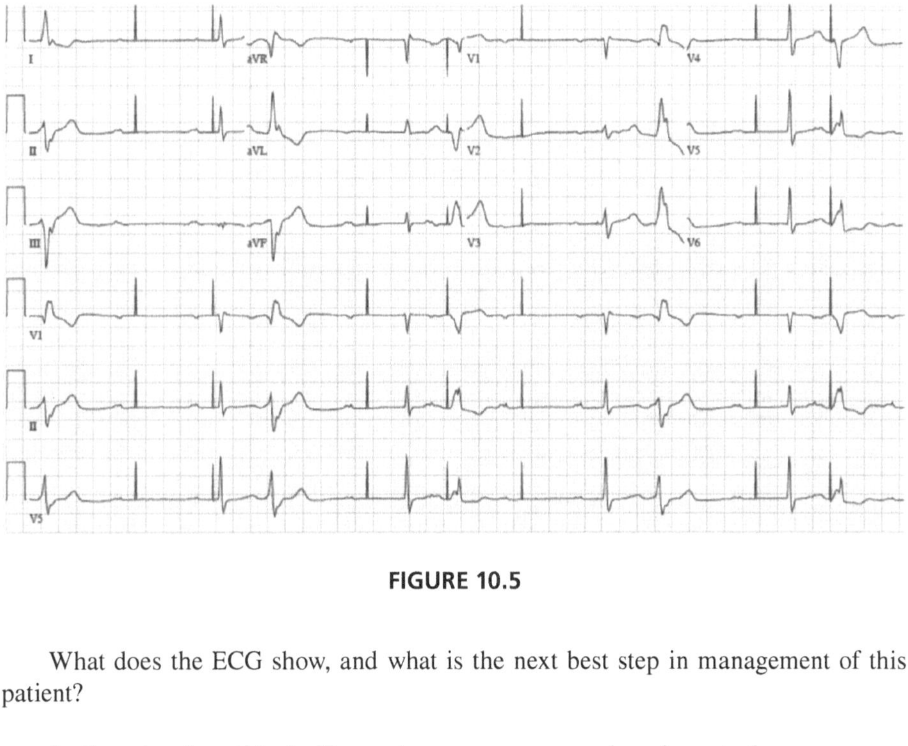

FIGURE 10.5

What does the ECG show, and what is the next best step in management of this patient?

A. Complete heart block; Place a transvenous pacemaker via central access
B. Atrial fibrillation; Initiate a beta blocker and titrate to an HR of 60
C. Normal sinus rhythm; Consult the EP service to revise the malfunctioning lead
D. Normal sinus rhythm; Discharge the patient with a Holter monitor
E. Atrial flutter; Obtain a nuclear stress test and echocardiogram

Question 6

A 28-year-old female is transported to the emergency department after she reported palpitations while at work. She was in her normal state of health until 3 weeks ago, when she developed myalgias, fatigue, and low-grade fevers. Her symptoms have progressed and now also include lightheadedness and exertional dyspnea. The patient denies any prior medical history or any medication use. She reports a visit to upstate New York for kayaking and hiking approximately 3–4 weeks ago. She denied any tick bites. On her physical exam, there are no signs of rash or neurological abnormalities. Her cardiac exam is notable for ectopy, without any murmurs or gallops. An ECG was also obtained, as seen below.

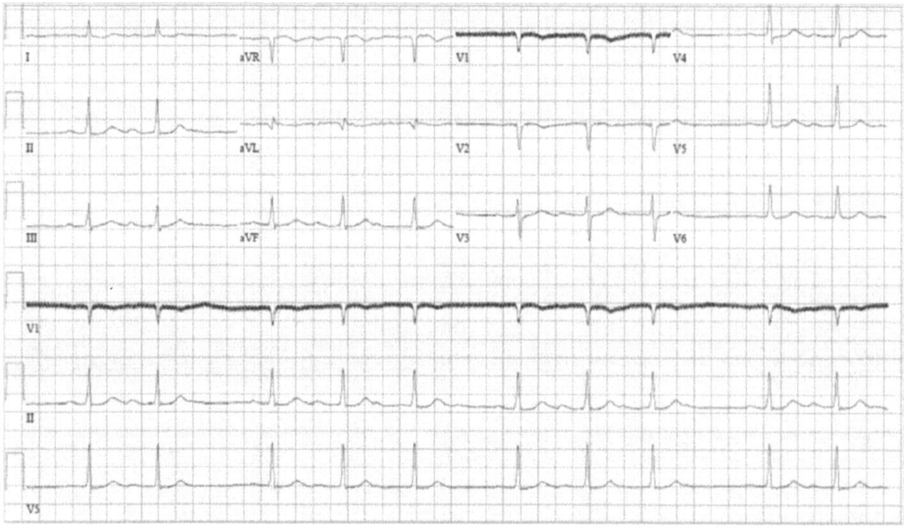

FIGURE 10.6

What does the ECG show, and is the appropriate pharmacotherapy for this patient?

A. 2nd degree AV Block, Type I; Intravenous Piperacillin-tazobactam
B. Complete heart block; Intravenous ampicillin-sulbactam
C. 2nd degree AV Block, Type II; Oral doxycycline
D. 2nd degree AV Block, Type I; Intravenous ceftriaxone
E. 2nd degree AV Block, Type II; Intramuscular penicillin

Question 7

A 41-year-old African–American male presents to the emergency department, describing acute chest pain that began this morning. He describes the pain as tightness and is associated with shortness of breath upon deep inspiration. He denies orthopnea, paroxysmal nocturnal dyspnea, lower extremity swelling, nausea, and syncope. He does endorse an upper respiratory infection that he had 3 weeks ago. His vitals are within normal limits. His physical exam reveals a normal cardiac exam with no rubs. CXR is without abnormalities. His ECG is shown below.

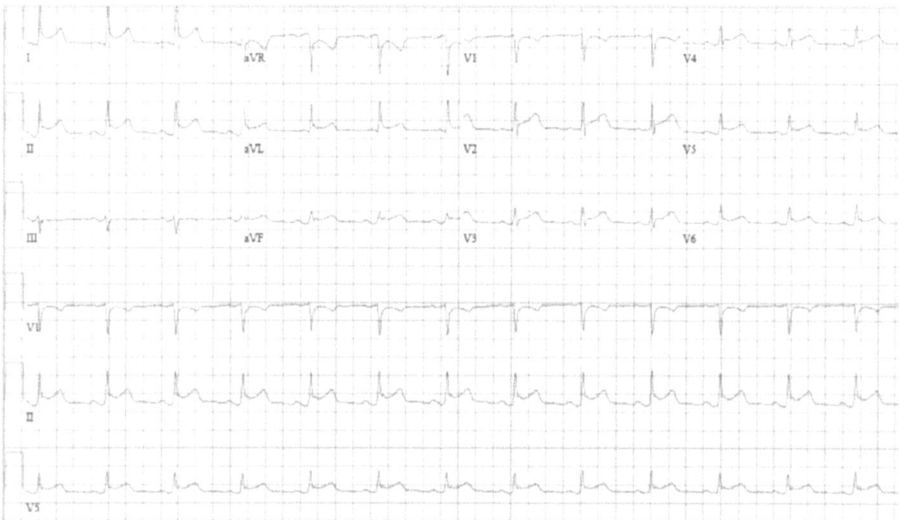

FIGURE 10.7

Which of the following answer choices pairs the correct ECG interpretation with the correct management?

A. STEMI; Load with aspirin, and activate the STEMI protocol
B. STEMI; Complete the tPA checklist and administer the medication
C. NSTEMI Type II; Start the patient on broad-spectrum antibiotics for pneumonia
D. Pericarditis; Order NSAIDs for pain control and colchicine as an anti-inflammatory
E. Pericarditis; Obtain an echocardiogram and perform a pericardiocentesis for fluid analysis

Question 8

A 55-year-old Caucasian female with no prior medical history presents to the primary care clinic as a new patient. She recently had her blood pressure checked at a health fair, which revealed multiple elevated BP measurements. The patient offers no complaints, and her review of systems is negative. Her vitals, which were repeated on both arms, were found to range 120–128/76–82. Her BMI is 24. The remainder of her exam is unremarkable. Her ECG is shown below.

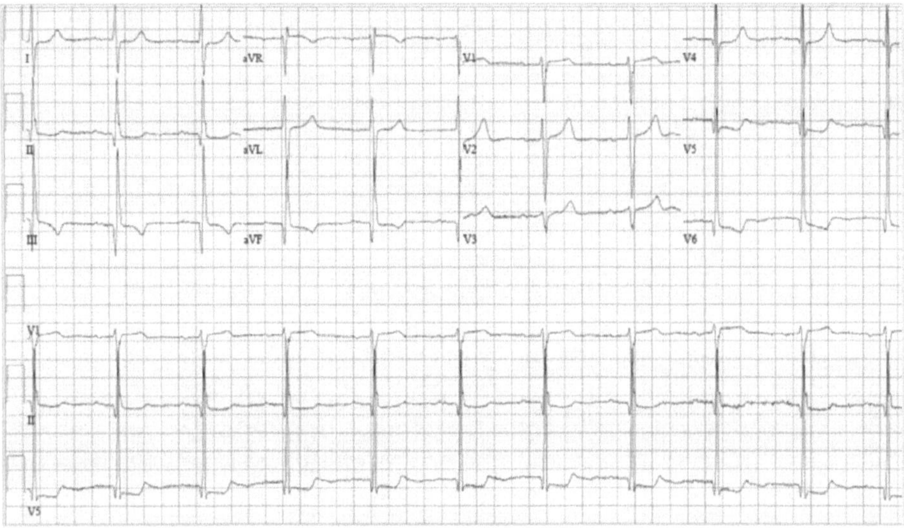

FIGURE 10.8

What does the ECG show, and what is the next best test to order?

A. Left ventricular hypertrophy; Plasma renin and aldosterone levels
B. Right ventricular hypertrophy; Renal ultrasound with arterial duplex
C. Right ventricular Hypertrophy; Sleep study to evaluate for obstructive sleep apnea
D. Biventricular hypertrophy; Serum metanephrines and normetanephrines
E. Left ventricular hypertrophy; 24-hour ambulatory blood pressure monitoring

Question 9

A 69-year-old African American male presents to his primary care clinic for a post-hospital discharge visit. He was admitted to a local community hospital for a myocardial infarction. He states to have had a prolonged hospital stay because he received a medication by EMS that made his blood pressure drop precipitously low. Since his discharge 4 days ago, he is symptom-free and has not had any chest pain, palpitations, shortness of breath, or peripheral edema. An ECG is obtained to determine the most likely culprit artery.

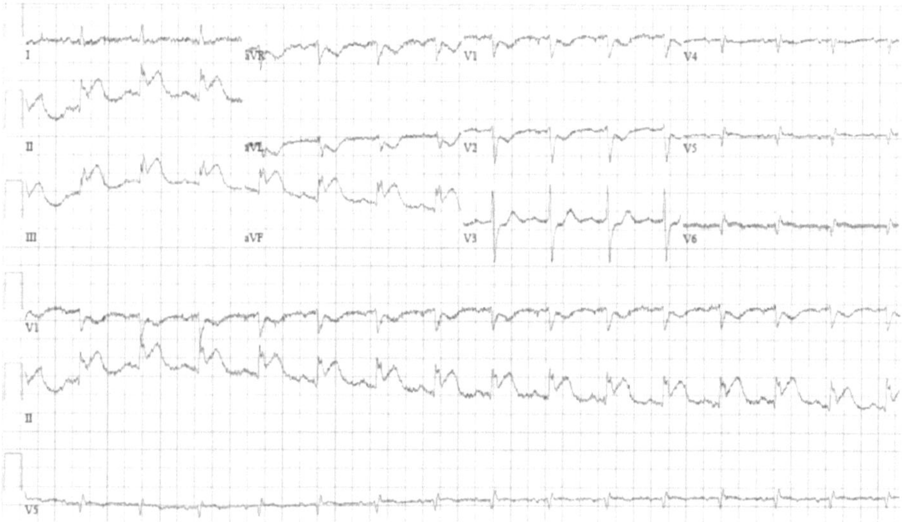

FIGURE 10.9

Which of the following answers pairs the correct ECG interpretation with the correct coronary artery?

A. Anterior STEMI; Left circumflex coronary artery
B. Inferior STEMI; Right coronary artery
C. Lateral STEMI; Left anterior descending coronary artery
D. Anterolateral STEMI; Right posterior descending coronary artery
E. Inferior STEMI; Left main coronary artery

Question 10

An 84-year-old Caucasian male with medical history of hypertension, diabetes on oral hypoglycemic medications, end-stage renal disease on dialysis, and multiple myeloma is sent from his Oncology Clinic to the emergency room for evaluation of altered mental status. His finger-stick glucose upon patient intake was mildly elevated. The patient complains of fatigue and palpitations. The patient admits to being non-adherent with his medications and dialysis sessions this week. In addition to labs, an ECG was obtained in the emergency department; the ECG is shown below.

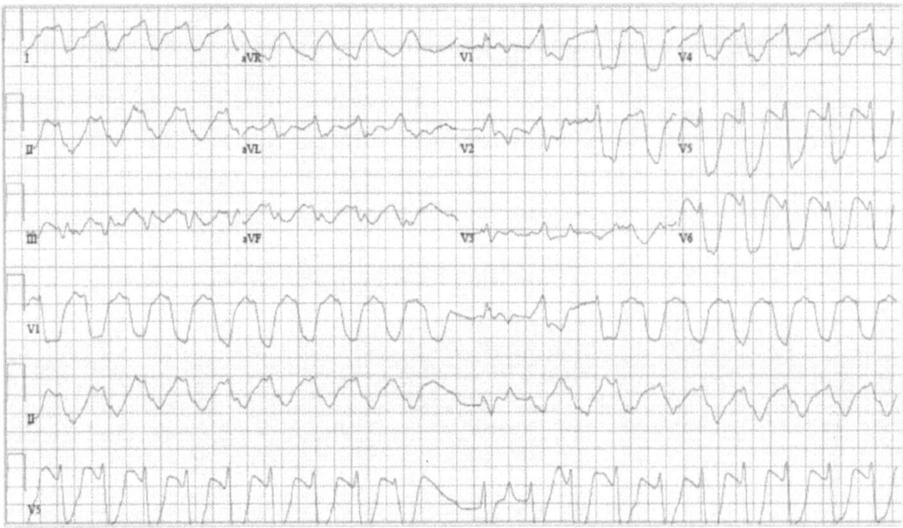

FIGURE 10.10

Which of the following matches the correct ECG interpretation to the correct management?

A. Torsades to Pointes; Order an insulin drip
B. QT Prolongation; Order a repeat set of labs
C. Hyperkalemia; Order calcium gluconate
D. Supraventricular Tachycardia; Order a bolus of Ringer's Lactate
E. Ventricular Tachycardia; Obtain an electrophysiology-cardiology consultation

Question 11

A 75-year-old African American female presents for routine follow-up of her chronic medical conditions. She has a past medical history of coronary artery disease having had an LAD stent placed a few years ago, hypertension, diabetes, and hypothyroidism. She takes her medications as prescribed (metoprolol, lisinopril, aspirin, atorvastatin, and levothyroxine). On physical exam, her vitals are all within normal limits, and her cardiac exam is noteworthy for an irregularly irregular rhythm. Her ECG obtained in clinic is shown below.

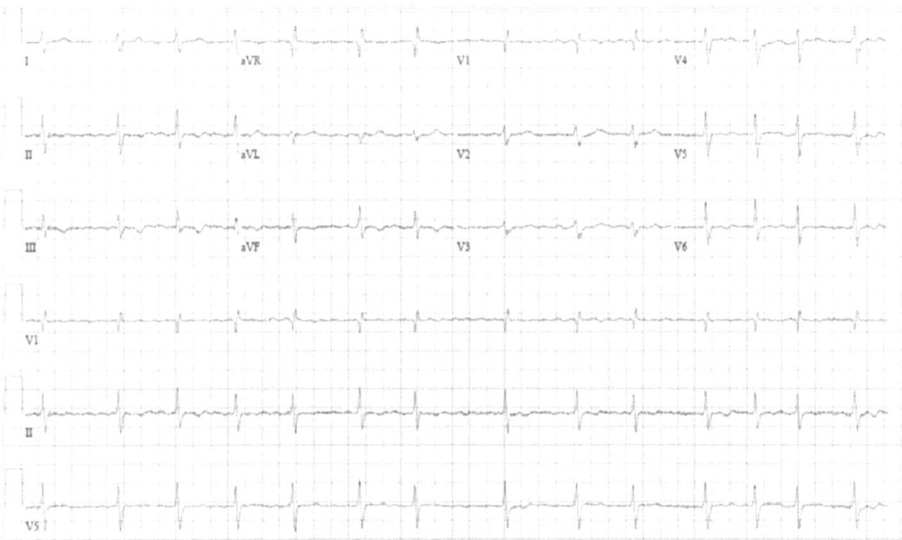

FIGURE 10.11

Which of the following matches the correct ECG interpretation to the correct management?

A. Atrial fibrillation; Continue aspirin, and start the patient on anticoagulation
B. Atrial flutter; Obtain an echocardiogram
C. Atrial fibrillation; Switch metoprolol to diltiazem
D. Atrial flutter; Add clopidogrel to her current medications
E. Atrial fibrillation; Discontinue aspirin and schedule the patient for a left atrial appendage occlusion

Question 12

An 83-year-old Spanish-speaking male with history of hypertension, gout, and obesity presents to the emergency room for an episode of syncope while eating dinner. He has developed fatigue and somnolence since the event. His wife, who accompanied him to the ED states this is uncharacteristic of her husband, who is usually very active. His physical exam reveals no pallor or dry mucous membranes, lungs clear to auscultation, and no thyromegaly appreciated. His cardiac exam is significant for a regular rhythm with faint holosystolic murmur. His ECG is shown below.

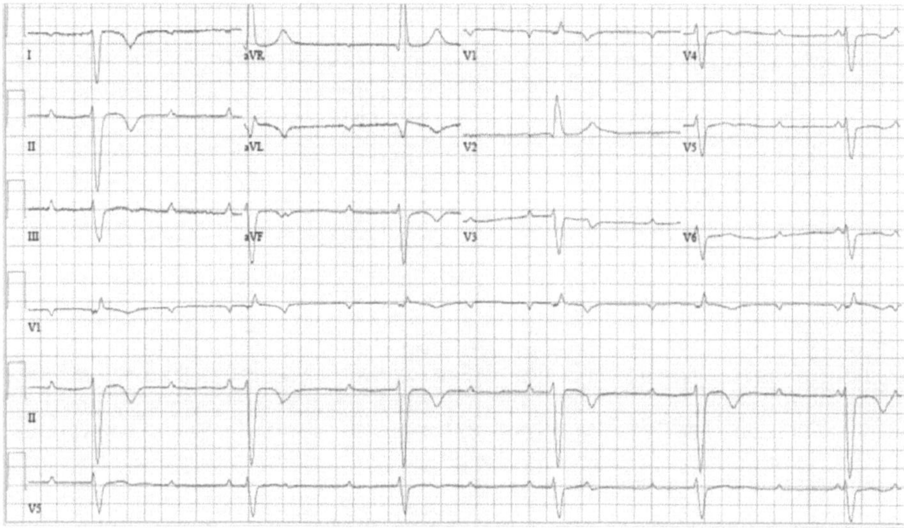

FIGURE 10.12

What is the next appropriate step in management?

A. 2nd degree AV Block, Mobitz I; Discontinue metoprolol
B. Complete Heart Block; Placement of transvenous pacer wire and plan for permanent pacemaker
C. Sinus Bradycardia; Discharge with close cardiology follow-up
D. 2nd degree AV Block, Mobitz II; Electrophysiology study for possible ICD implantation
E. 2nd degree AV Block, Mobitz II; Echocardiography to evaluate systolic murmur heard on exam

Question 13

A 42-year-old Asian American male who recently suffered a meniscal injury of the left knee presents for evaluation prior to an elective arthroscopic procedure. His only medical history is hypertension, for which he takes losartan. His review of systems is negative for chest pain, palpitations, and exertional dyspnea. His vitals are all normal. His physical exam is unremarkable, aside from a limited range of motion in his left knee. His ECG is shown below.

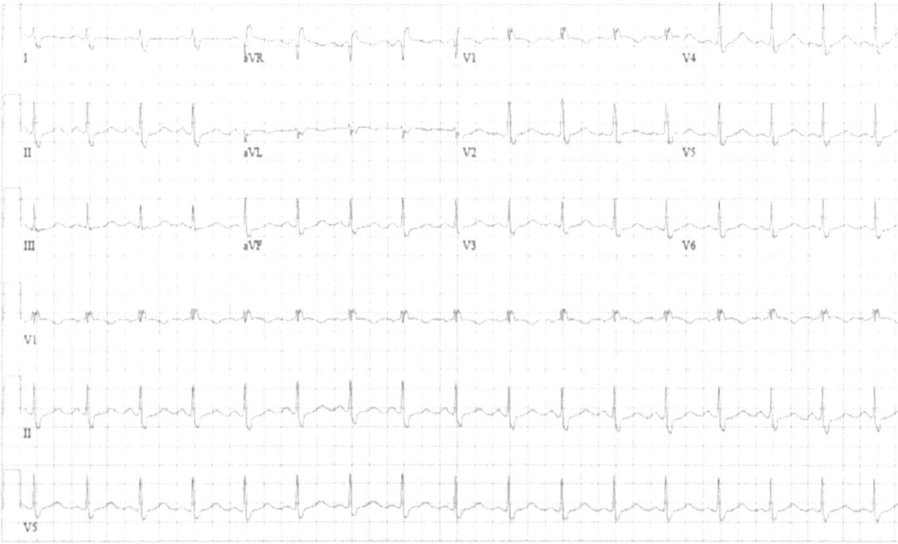

FIGURE 10.13

What does the ECG show, and what is the next best step in management?

A. Incomplete RBBB; No further testing is indicated
B. RBBB; Referral to cardiology for further evaluation
C. J-point elevation; Chemical nuclear stress testing
D. Incomplete LBBB; Echocardiography
E. LBBB; Prophylactic pacemaker implantation

Question 14

A 57-year-old Bangladeshi-American female with a medical history of hypertension presented to the emergency room for stroke-like symptoms. Her presenting symptoms were right-sided hemiparesis, which resolved within 24 hours of admission. A CT scan of the head demonstrated multiple, small acute strokes. Her ECG is shown below. Her transthoracic echocardiogram with bubble study was negative for a patent foramen ovale and unremarkable from a structural standpoint. The ultrasound of her carotids shows <30% stenosis and was deemed unlikely to be the etiology of her stroke. Telemetry has shown no arrhythmias during her hospital stay. The patient was started on a statin and aspirin during this admission. The patient is now medically stable for discharge.

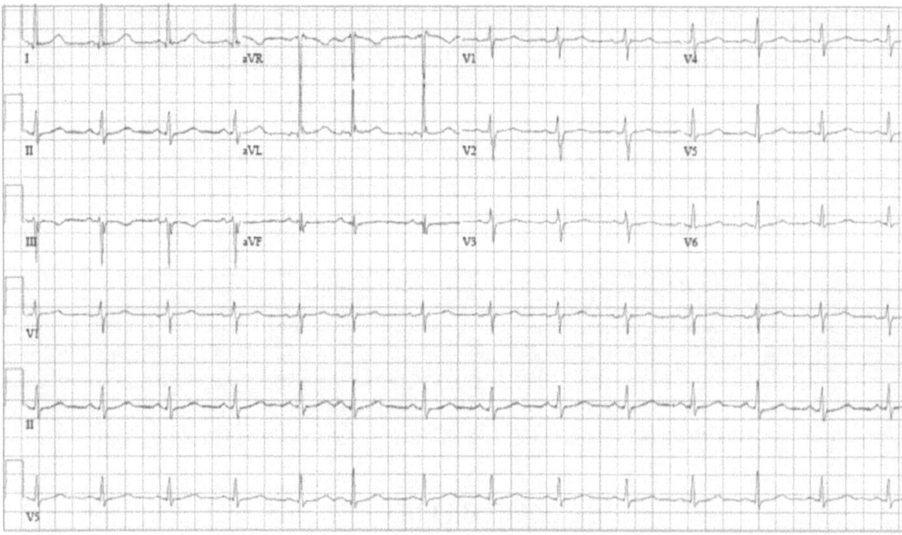

FIGURE 10.14

Which of the following should be done prior to discharge?

A. Send off a hypercoagulability work-up and encourage outpatient follow-up
B. Place an implantable loop recorder to evaluate for episodes of atrial fibrillation
C. Referral to outpatient cardiologist for elective cardiac catheterization
D. Order an outpatient PET scan for occult malignancy and encourage outpatient follow-up
E. Prescription for MRI of the spine to evaluate for demyelinating disease and neurology follow-up

Question 15

A 34-year-old male with a medical history of hypertension is evaluated in the emergency department after suffering a fall from standing height and landing on his left chest wall. At present, he endorses mild musculoskeletal chest discomfort that is reproducible upon palpation of his chest wall. A CT scan of the chest reveals subcutaneous edema overlying the left chest wall but no fractures, dislocations, or lacerations. An echocardiogram is obtained and is unremarkable. He is placed on telemetry monitoring, and an ECG is obtained (shown below). The patient is an avid marathon runner and asks the physician if it is safe for him to continue training.

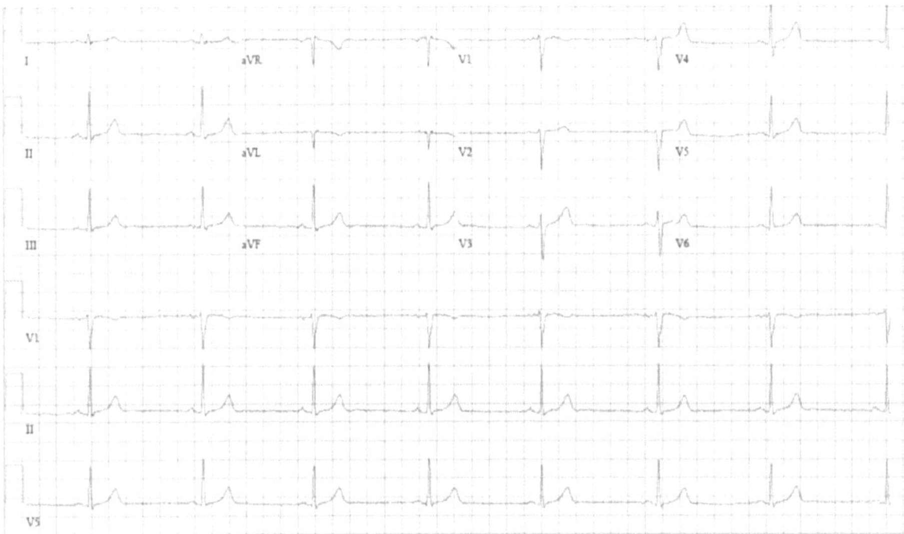

FIGURE 10.15

What does the ECG show, and which of the following responses is most appropriate for the patient's question?

A. Sinus Bradycardia; "Your heart rate is too slow and requires further evaluation with a cardiologist"
B. Normal Sinus Rhythm; "Performing any strenuous activity is forbidden, given your recent fall"
C. Normal Sinus Rhythm; "You should hold off on running in a marathon because you have chest pain"
D. Sinus Bradycardia; "I will prescribe you a baby aspirin to take daily because of your history of hypertension"
E. Sinus Bradycardia; "Your heart appears normal, and you can resume training for the marathon when you feel ready"

Question 16

A 67-year-old male with a medical history of hypertension, dyslipidemia, type 2 diabetes mellitus, hyperthyroidism, and generalized anxiety disorder presents to the emergency department complaining of LLQ abdominal pain. The patient appears anxious and reports that the pain has prevented him from eating and drinking. His vital signs are noteworthy for a temperature of 38.0 degrees Celsius and a heart rate of 115 BPM. The patient has an IV line placed and is sent to the CT scanner. The results demonstrate diverticulitis within the descending colon, and antibiotics are promptly started. An ECG performed upon admission is shown below.

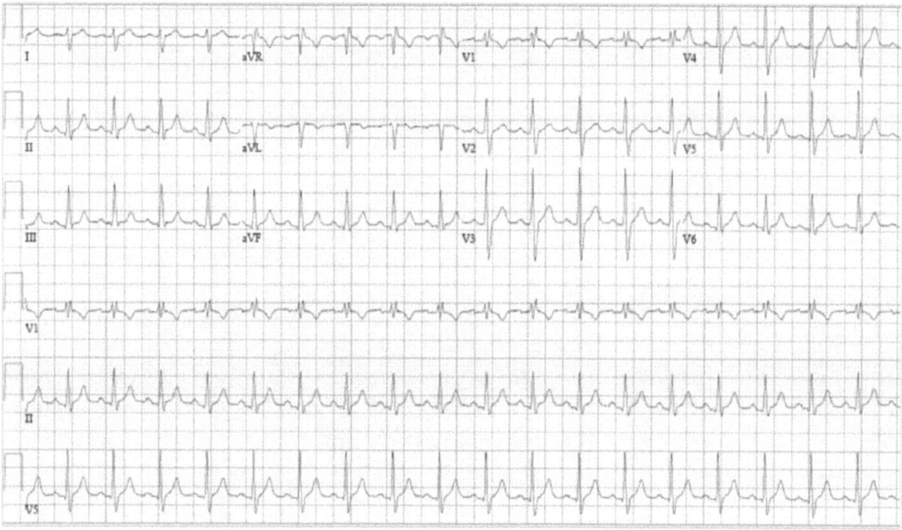

FIGURE 10.16

What does the ECG show, and which of the following pharmacotherapies would NOT be appropriate at this time?

A. Sinus Tachycardia; Alprazolam
B. Sinus Tachycardia; Metoprolol
C. Sinus Tachycardia; Normal Saline bolus
D. Ectopic Atrial Rhythm; Acetaminophen
E. Normal Sinus Rhythm; Morphine

Question 17

A 20-year-old male comes to your primary care clinic to establish care after his pediatrician retired. He recently participated in a CPR-certification class, and his instructor performed an ECG to demonstrate how the equipment worked. His instructor notified the patient after the class that he noticed "ST changes" on the monitor and recommended that the patient sees his doctor to have a formal ECG performed. The patient reports that his heart will occasionally "skip a beat," but that it rarely occurs and is not associated with chest pain, shortness of breath, or any other cardiac symptoms. His vital signs, physical exam, and labs are unremarkable. The nurse is called in, and the ECG obtained is displayed below.

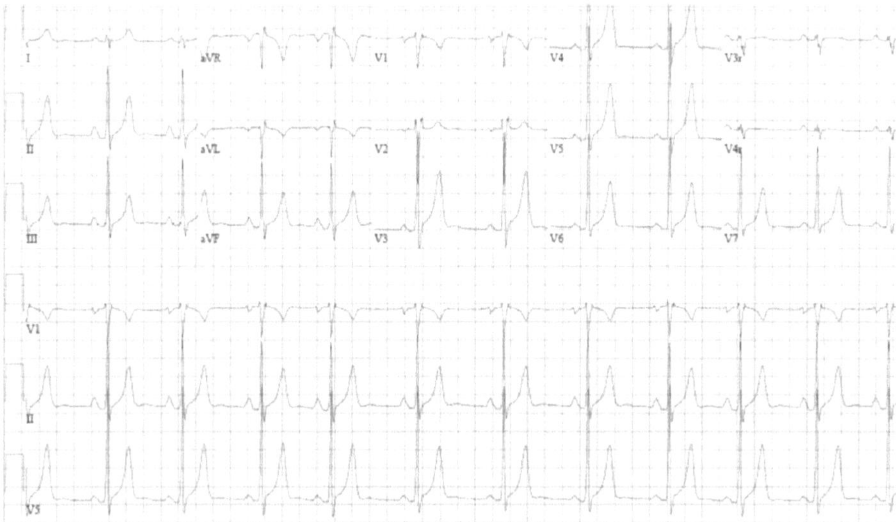

FIGURE 10.17

Which of the following matches the correct ECG interpretation with the correct management?

A. J-point elevation; refer the patient to the ED
B. Delta wave; refer the patient for an urgent EP study
C. Early repolarization; provide reassurance
D. Brugada Syndrome; refer the patient for an urgent ICD implantation
E. 1st Degree AV Block; provide reassurance

Question 18

An 84-year-old Hispanic female with a past medical history of hypertension, type 2 diabetes mellitus, dyslipidemia, and colonic angiodysplasia presents to the emergency department complaining of hematochezia. She is given 1 unit of packed red blood cells for anemia. Her vital signs are all within normal limits. The GI team recommends a bowel preparation and a colonoscopy in the morning. However, a 2/4 diastolic murmur with an opening snap is heard at the apex during cardiac auscultation. An echocardiogram is scheduled, and an ECG (shown below) is obtained. The patient reported that she had "bad infection" when she was a child and, as a result, developed a "valve problem."

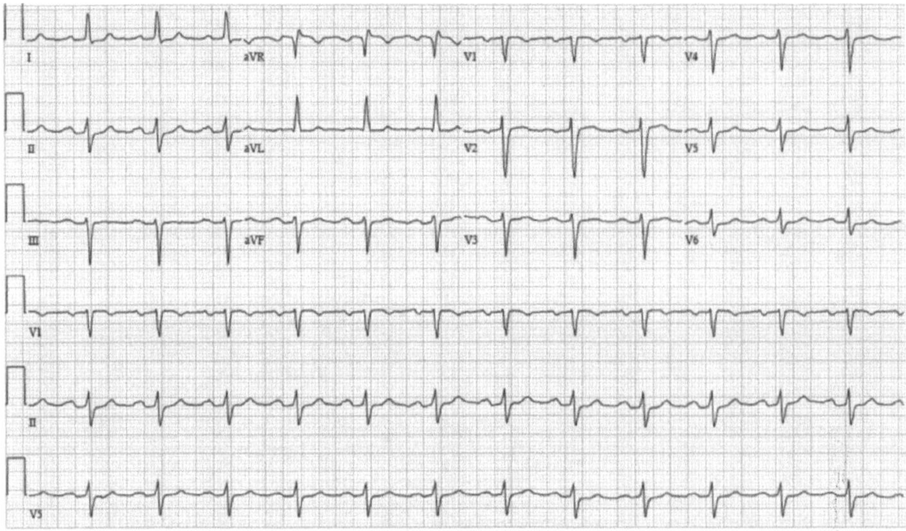

FIGURE 10.18

Which of the following findings on the ECG is consistent with the patient's history and cardiac auscultation?

A. Widened P-waves > 120 ms in duration
B. Tall P-waves in Lead V1 > 1.5 mm
C. Widened QRS > 120 ms in duration
D. Tall R-wave in Lead aVL > 11 mm
E. Upright QRS complexes in Leads I and II

Question 19

A 71-year-old African-American male with a past medical history of recent pulmonary embolism on apixaban and high-grade atrioventricular block status post-PPM implantation is scheduled for an elective TEE/cardioversion for new-onset atrial fibrillation noted on remote monitoring. The patient has been mostly adherent with his apixaban as an outpatient but missed a few doses in the past 30 days. He endorses feeling palpitations but denies other cardiac symptoms. His pre-cardioversion ECG demonstrates atrial fibrillation. After the TEE rules out thrombus within the left atrial appendage and demonstrates no significant valvular heart disease, the electrical cardioversion is performed. The patient's post-cardioversion ECG is shown below. After awakening from anesthesia, the patient reports that he feels well and is looking forward to being released.

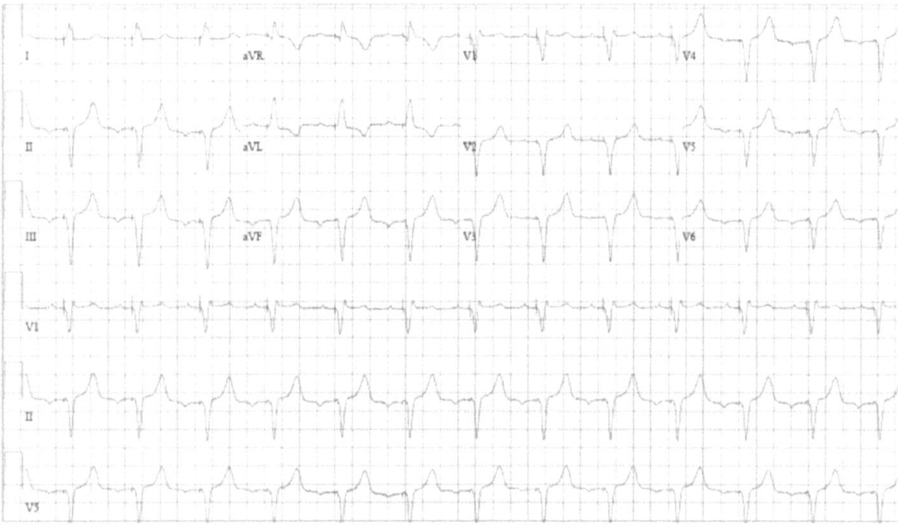

FIGURE 10.19

Which of the following is the correct interpretation of the ECG?

A. Normal sinus rhythm, without ventricular pacing
B. Ectopic atrial rhythm, without ventricular pacing
C. Normal sinus rhythm, with ventricular pacing
D. Ectopic atrial rhythm, with ventricular pacing
E. Normal sinus rhythm, with atrioventricular sequential pacing

Question 20

An 85-year-old Spanish-speaking male with a past medical history of mild cognitive impairment and hypertension presents to the cardiology clinic for a routine visit. He had previously been referred to a cardiologist months earlier when he was diagnosed with symptomatic atrial fibrillation. He underwent a cardioversion without complications and had been in normal sinus rhythm ever since. The patient has an ECG performed in the cardiology clinic, which is displayed below. The patient denies chest pain, palpitations, shortness of breath, dyspnea on exertion, and presyncope. His vital signs and most recent blood work are unremarkable.

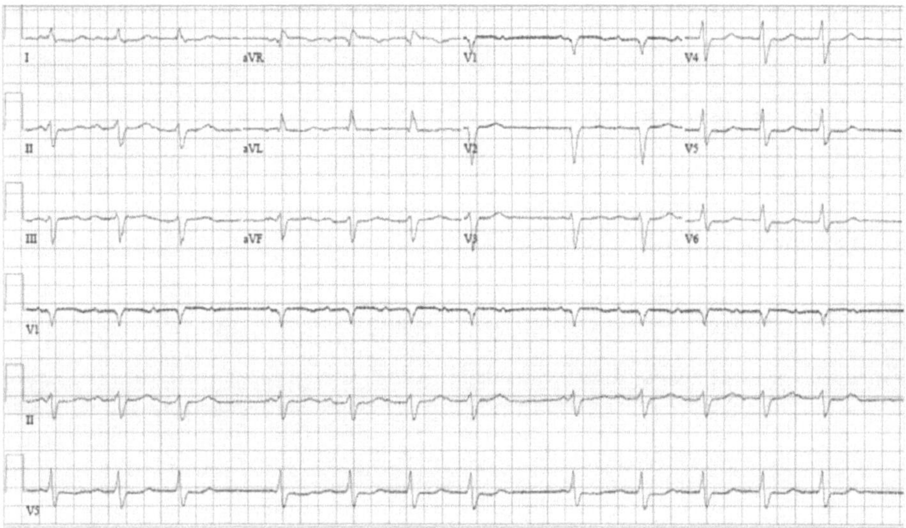

FIGURE 10.20

Which of the following pairs is the correct ECG interpretation to the correct management?

A. 2nd degree AV Block, Mobitz II; Administer atropine IM and observe for an improvement in his heart rate
B. 2nd degree AV Block, Mobitz I; Refer the patient to the ED for admission to a cardiac unit
C. 2nd degree AV Block, Mobitz II; Schedule the patient for a permanent pacemaker implantation
D. 2nd degree AV Block, Mobitz II; Test the patient for Lyme disease with a serum PCR
E. 2nd degree AV Block, Mobitz I; Provide reassurance, as the rhythm is not causing symptoms

Question 21

A 76-year-old Caucasian female with a medical history of hypertension, peripheral vascular disease, and hyperlipidemia presents to the emergency department for a sensation of intermittent palpitations and presyncope. An ECG is performed, and the results are shown below. The patient is admitted to the cardiology unit for further work-up, and placed on telemetry. While on telemetry, tracings similar to those found on the ECG are evident. She asks what the next steps are while she is admitted.

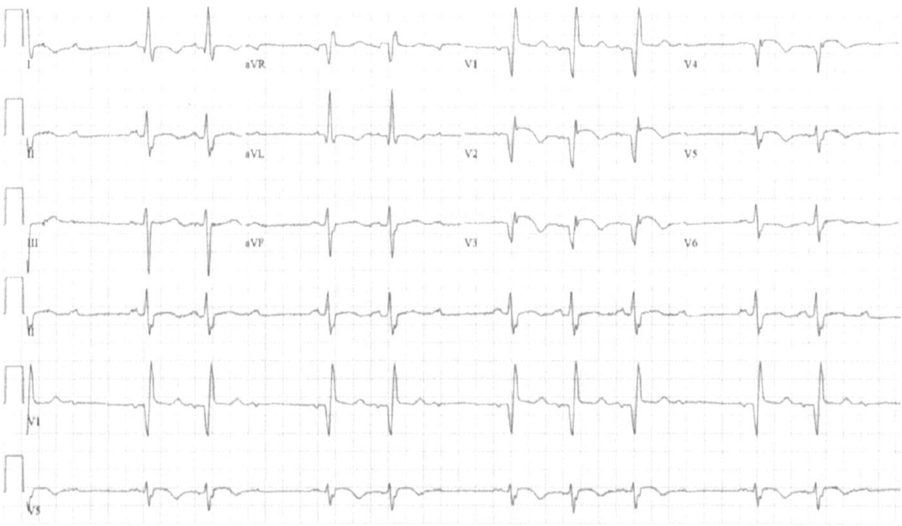

FIGURE 10.21

What does the ECG show, and which of the following is the best response to this patient?

A. NSR; "Because your palpitations are so infrequent, you can be discharged today with a Holter monitor"
B. 2nd Degree AV Block, Mobitz II; "The pauses on your ECG warrant a pacemaker, irrespective of symptoms"
C. Sinus Pauses; "You will need to have an ICD implanted due to the risk of the pauses causing cardiac arrest"
D. PVCs; "You will need to be discharged on a beta blocker to decrease the frequency of these palpitations"
E. 2nd Degree AV Block, Mobitz I; "The abnormalities on your ECG are common in patients your age; no treatment is required"

Question 22

An 82-year-old Spanish-speaking female is brought to the emergency department due to a witnessed fall. The patient has a past medical history of hypertension, hypothyroidism, iron deficiency anemia, osteoarthritis, and pre-diabetes. The patient's daughter reports that the patient had been feeling weak for the past 2–3 days. She saw her mother "get woozy," lose consciousness, and then fall while sitting in a chair. She was able to catch the patient before she fell to the ground. There was no seizure-like activity after the patient lost consciousness. The patient had normal vital signs, and orthostatic vital signs were negative. There were no murmurs on cardiac auscultation, but her ECG (shown below) concerned the providers in the ED.

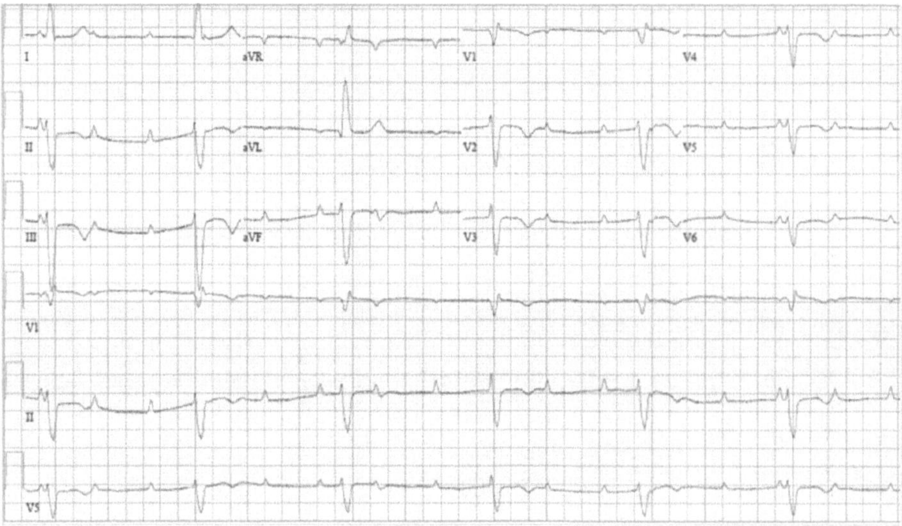

FIGURE 10.22

Which of the following pairs the correct ECG interpretation with the correct management?

A. 2nd degree AV Block, Mobitz II; Schedule an inpatient permanent pacemaker implantation
B. Complete heart block; Place a transvenous pacing wire prior to implanting a permanent pacemaker
C. Normal sinus rhythm; Consult hematology urgently for further work-up and administer IV iron sulfate
D. 2nd degree AV Block, Mobitz I; Obtain an echocardiogram to rule out a valvular etiology of her syncope
E. Atrial fibrillation; Place the patient on a 24-hour video EEG and obtain an MRI of the brain

Question 23

A 69-year-old Caucasian male presents to the ED in December complaining of worsening shortness of breath. The patient talks with some conversational dyspnea but can report that he has a history of emphysema and hypertension. He endorses receiving his "pneumonia vaccines," as well as his annual flu vaccine, 2 weeks earlier. The ECG that was obtained by providers in the ED is shown below. The patient denies any heart problems or a history of arrhythmias. His blood work is notable for an elevated WCC with a lymphocytic predominance and a respiratory viral panel that was positive for rhinovirus. A CT angiogram of the chest was performed, which ruled out a pulmonary embolism.

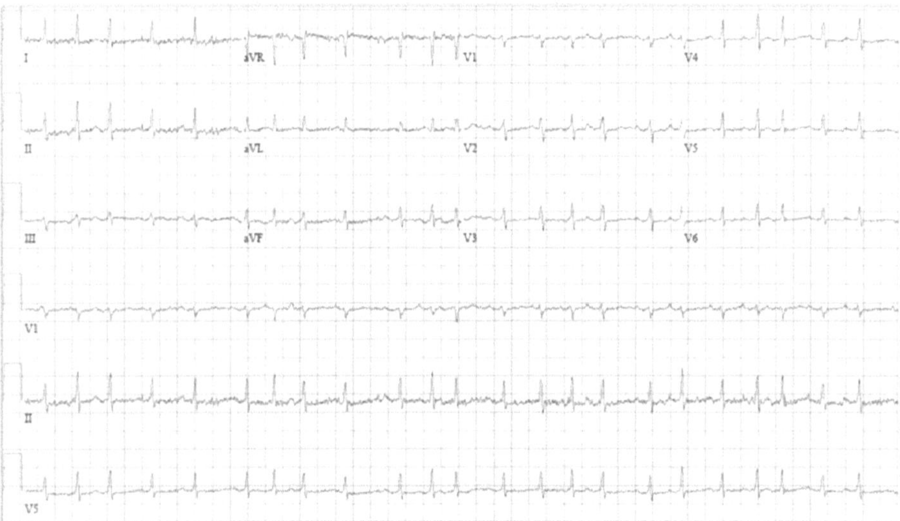

FIGURE 10.23

What does the ECG show, and which of the following is the most appropriate management of the arrhythmia?

A. Atrial fibrillation; Initiate a heparin drip or subcutaneous enoxaparin
B. Multifocal atrial tachycardia; Perform an echocardiogram to evaluate for wall motion abnormalities
C. Multifocal atrial tachycardia; Provide supportive care for the COPD exacerbation
D. Atrial fibrillation; Initiate metoprolol tartrate by mouth, with a goal of HR <110 BPM
E. Atrial flutter with aberrant conduction; Schedule the patient for a TEE/ cardioversion

Question 24

A 40-year-old African American male presents to the hospital due to palpitations and lightheadedness. The patient reports that he began feeling these symptoms yesterday morning after he awoke. He denies any history of heart problems, as well as any past medical history. When asked about his social history, he responded that he did "over-indulge" at a party two nights ago, drinking eight mixed alcoholic drinks. The patient is placed on telemetry and given injection of diltiazem before a formal ECG (shown below) is obtained. While on telemetry, he spontaneously converts back to normal sinus rhythm. The patient asks if blood thinners will be needed in the long term to prevent him from having a stroke.

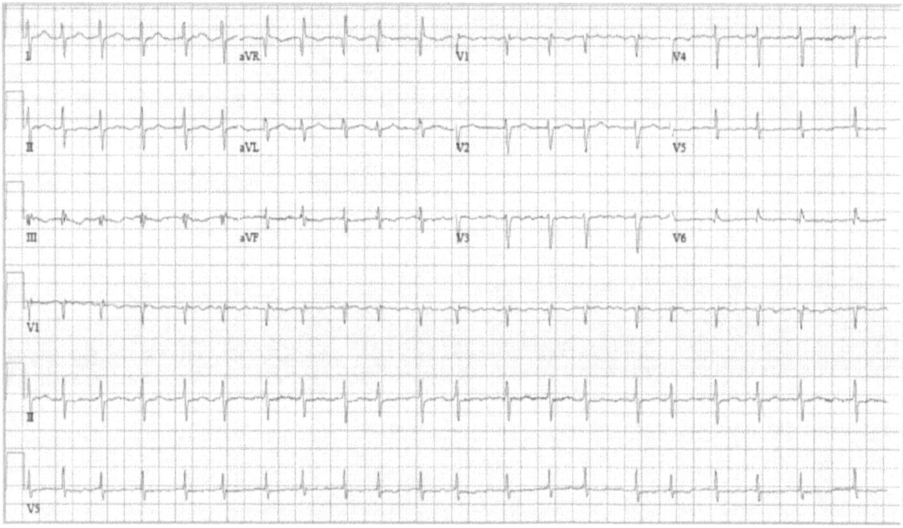

FIGURE 10.24

Which of the following is the most appropriate answer to give the patient?

A. "Your CHA_2DS_2VASc Score is 0, so aspirin is indicated"
B. "Your CHA_2DS_2VASc Score is 1 due to your sex, so aspirin is indicated"
C. "Your CHA_2DS_2VASc Score is 2 due to your sex and ethnicity, so anticoagulation is indicated"
D. "Your CHA_2DS_2VASc Score is 1 due to your sex, so anticoagulation is indicated"
E. "Your CHA_2DS_2VASc Score is 0, so no aspirin or anticoagulation is indicated"

Question 25

A 77-year-old Caucasian female presents to the emergency department complaining of shortness of breath and fatigue for the past 2 weeks. She has a history of hypertension, hypothyroidism, COPD, and panic disorder. She denies any cardiac history or use of blood thinners, but does report that she had a "sonogram of [her] heart" and ECG last year for shortness of breath, which demonstrated a normal ejection fraction and normal sinus rhythm. She also completed PFTs, which were consistent with obstructive lung disease. A full panel of TFTs ordered by her endocrinologist was unremarkable. The ECG obtained in the ED is displayed below.

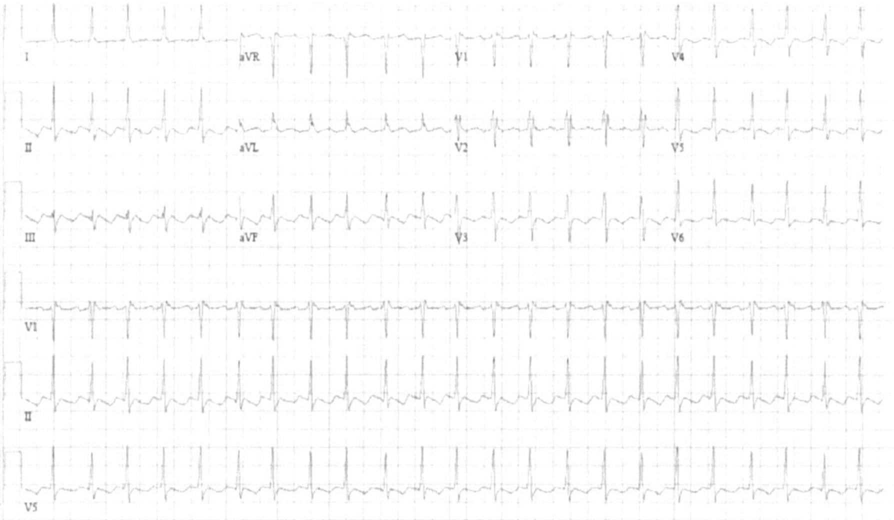

FIGURE 10.25

Given the above, which of the following medications would be LEAST preferred to control her arrhythmia at this time?

A. Metoprolol
B. Digoxin
C. Amiodarone
D. Diltiazem
E. Magnesium

Question 26

A 50-year-old African–American female presents to the hospital with palpitations. She reports that she has no past medical history but does admit that she has not seen a doctor since she delivered her second child 17 years ago. Her only medication is a multivitamin. Her heart rate per telemetry monitoring shows a constant rate of 138 BPM. An ED provider is concerned for an arrhythmia and obtains the ECG displayed below. The remaining work-up, including CXR and blood work, is unremarkable.

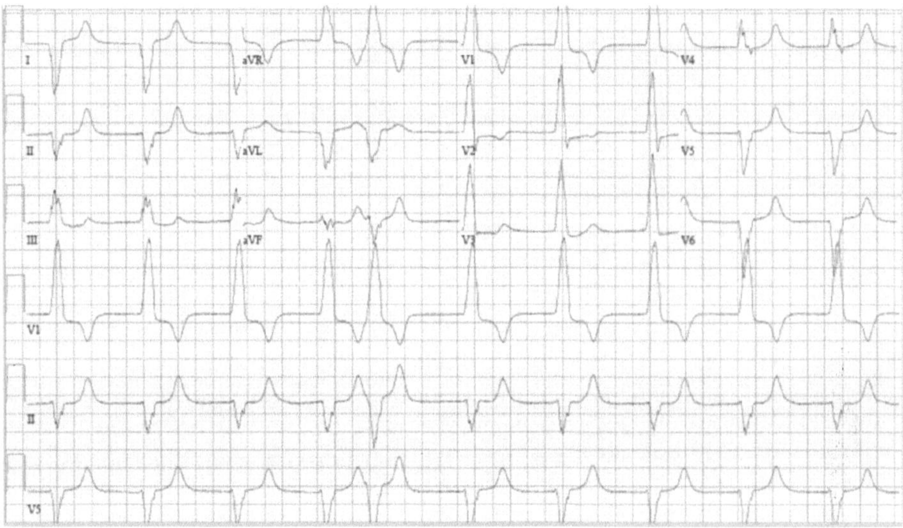

FIGURE 10.26

Which of the following is TRUE about the arrhythmia pictured in the ECG?

A. F-waves classically have different morphologies within the same lead
B. Ablation always has a high success rate in treating atrial fibrillation
C. The focus for typical atrial flutter is the cavotricuspid isthmus
D. Atrial flutter rarely develops because of cardiac surgery, unlike atrial fibrillation
E. Anticoagulation is not required for atrial flutter due to the low risk of thromboembolism

Question 27

A 70-year-old Asian male with a medical history of dextrocardia, CAD, peripheral vascular disease, and hypertension presented to the emergency department, complaining of chest pain. Earlier in the day, the patient developed a crushing pressure over his chest while shoveling snow. After calling 911, he took 325 mg of aspirin and 1 sublingual tab of nitroglycerin, which did not relieve the pain. Upon arrival at the ED, an ECG is performed, and a Code STEMI was called. The patient received two stents to his LAD and was placed in the cardiology unit for closer monitoring. Less than 1 hour after the cardiac catheterization was performed, telemetry showed an arrhythmia; the following ECG was obtained.

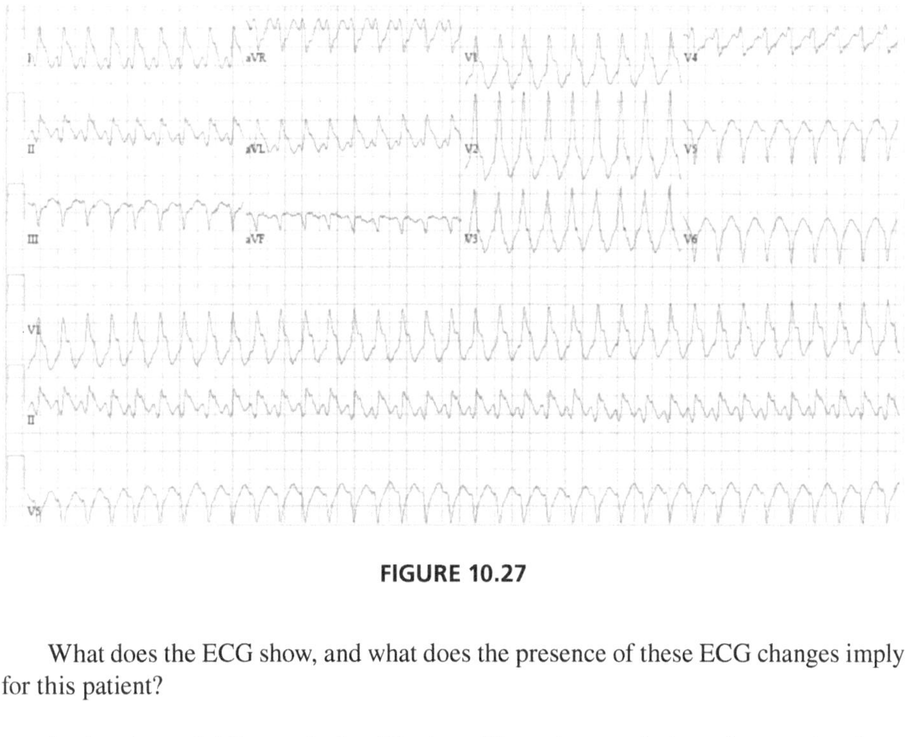

FIGURE 10.27

What does the ECG show, and what does the presence of these ECG changes imply for this patient?

A. Accelerated Idioventricular Rhythm; There is reperfusion of a previously occluded artery
B. Ventricular Tachycardia; There is in-stent re-thrombosis within the LAD
C. Ventricular Tachycardia; There is residual disease in another artery with ongoing ischemia
D. Junctional Escape Rhythm; There is SA nodal infarction, due to the lack of P-waves
E. Accelerated Idioventricular Rhythm; The arrhythmia is signaling an impending VT arrest

Question 28

An 85-year-old male with a past medical history of COPD on 2 Liters home oxygen, hypertension, dyslipidemia, and pre-diabetes presents to the ED with a cough productive of yellow-green sputum. He has a fever of 38.3 degrees Celsius, HR 107, BP 97/64, and a peripheral saturation of 91% on 2LNC. Blood work revealed an elevated WCC with a neutrophilic predominance. CXR revealed an RLL consolidation, concerning for pneumonia. The patient is started on ceftriaxone and azithromycin, haloperidol for delirium, as well as ondansetron for nausea. The following telemetry strip was obtained. Seconds later, the rhythm resolves, and the patient's vital signs normalize.

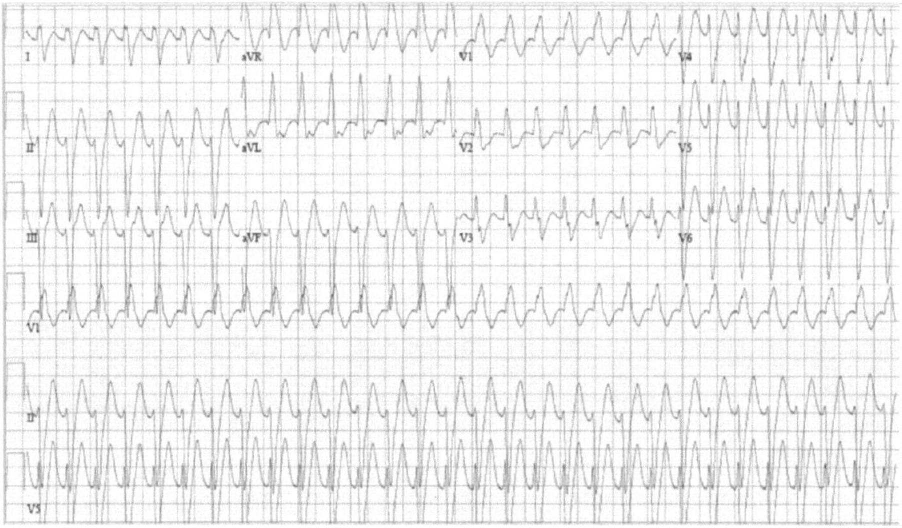

FIGURE 10.28

Which of the following pairs the correct ECG interpretation with the correct management?

A. Torsades de Pointes; Metoprolol infusion
B. Ventricular fibrillation; Isoproterenol infusion
C. Monomorphic ventricular tachycardia; Amiodarone infusion
D. Torsades de Pointes; Magnesium infusion
E. Supraventricular tachycardia; Vagal maneuvers

Question 29

A 79-year-old Caucasian female with a past medical history of CAD complicated by two STEMIs, atrial fibrillation on apixaban, hypertension, hyperlipidemia, and Sjogren's disease is admitted to the general medical floors for urosepsis. Shortly after admission, the patient began to complain of chest pain and lightheadedness. An ECG was performed immediately, which is shown below. On exam, the patient appeared uncomfortable but always maintained a palpable pulse. The responding team members were discussing whether the ECG represented SVT with aberrancy or ventricular tachycardia.

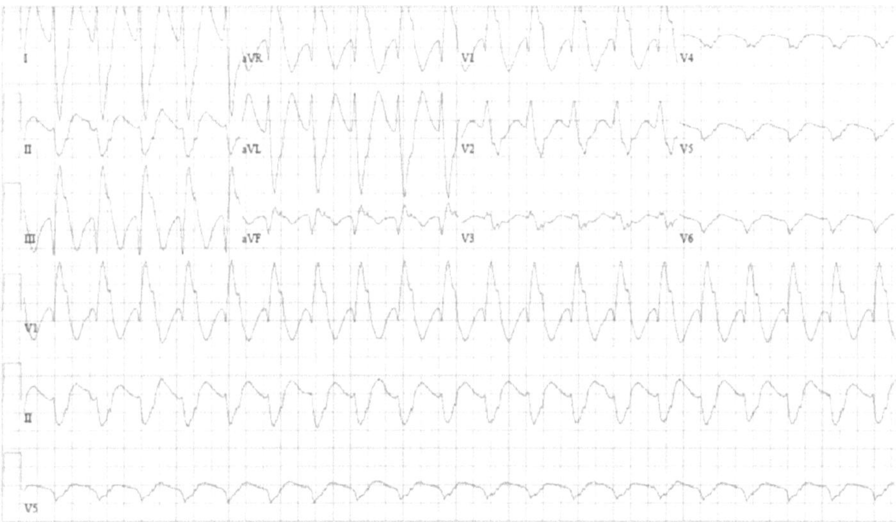

FIGURE 10.29

Which of the following characteristics are NOT part of the Brugada algorithm to delineate SVT from VT?

A. The presence of AV dissociation
B. The presence of inverted T-waves
C. The presence of an RS interval > 100 ms
D. The presence of LBBB/RBBB morphology in Lead V1
E. The absence of an RS interval in the precordial leads

Question 30

A 56-year-old Asian female with a past medical history of CAD, hypertension, hyperlipidemia, hypothyroidism, and pre-diabetes presents to the emergency room complaining of chest pain. The diagnosis of an inferior wall STEMI is made in the emergency department, and a Code STEMI is called. However, by the time the cardiology team arrives, the patient appears to be somnolent but arousable. In contrast to her ECG upon admission, which demonstrated sinus tachycardia with inferior wall ST-segment elevations, a repeat ECG is obtained (shown below).

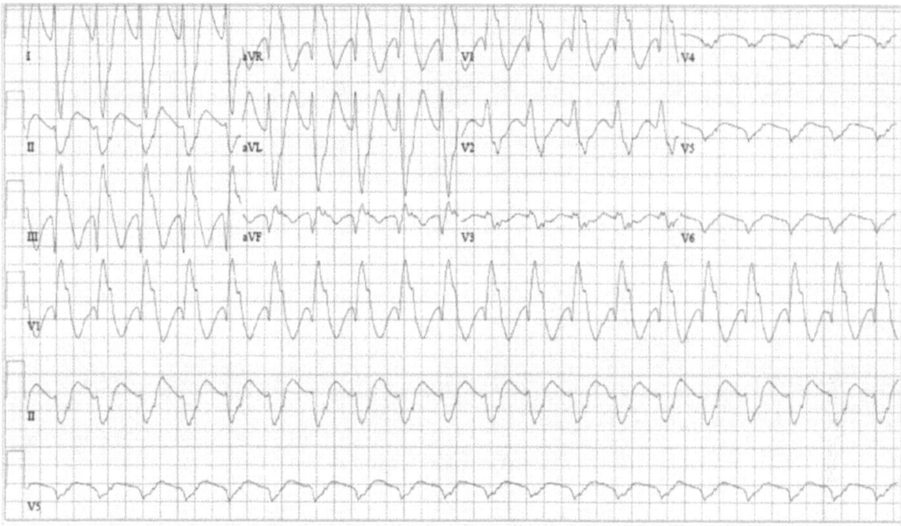

FIGURE 10.30

Which of the following pairs the correct ECG interpretation with the correct pharmacotherapy?

A. Ventricular fibrillation; epinephrine
B. Polymorphic VT; adenosine
C. Monomorphic VT; magnesium
D. Polymorphic VT; epinephrine
E. Monomorphic VT; amiodarone

OBJECTIVES AND ANSWERS

Q1. Identify new LBBB in patient with syncope without prodrome; appropriate referral to EPS for PPM

Answer: C

This patient has had multiple syncopal episodes without prodrome in the context of a new-onset LEFT bundle branch block. This is evident based upon the prolonged QRS complex (>120 ms in duration), with a characteristic dominant S-wave in V1, a broad monophasic R-wave in V6, and notching of the QRS within the lateral leads—all of which are present here. In the context of a new-onset LBBB, permanent pacing is indicated for unexplained syncope **(Choice C)**.

Q2. Recognize myocardial infarction (STEMI); appropriate therapy indicated for STEMI

Answer: B

This patient presents with chest pain, which is concerning for acute coronary syndrome. His ECG demonstrates the hallmarks of an acute anterolateral ST-elevation myocardial infarction (STEMI); he has >2 mm ST-segment elevations within the anterior (V2–V4) and lateral (I, V5, V6, and aVL) leads when compared with the TP segment, along with reciprocal depressions within the inferior leads (most notably in Lead III). In the case of a STEMI, a "STEMI protocol" involving revascularization should be activated **(Choice B)**.

Q3. Identify left atrial enlargement; associated with atrial fibrillation

Answer: A

The patient's ECG shows normal sinus rhythm but also has evidence of a left atrial abnormality (LAA). LAA is defined as the presence of a notched P-wave of >120 ms duration in the inferior leads (Lead II, III, or aVF) and may be a consequence of mitral valve disease, with or without a terminal negative deflection of the P-wave in Lead V1 that is >1 mm deep, and at least 40 ms in duration. Atrial fibrillation and LAA are associated with one another due to enlargement and damage to the atrial fibers, predisposing to arrhythmias **(Choice A)**.

Q4. Identify drug-induced prolonged QT; identify agents implicated in QT prolongation

Answer: C

This patient takes multiple QTc-prolonging medications, such as haloperidol, sertraline, and azithromycin. His ECG demonstrates QTc-prolongation, which is typically defined as a QTc interval greater than 450 ms in males. Even in patients who are asymptomatic, those with QTc-prolongation >500 ms should be considered for inpatient evaluation and telemetry monitoring. Regardless, offending medications should also be stopped or replaced, as this is likely contributing to the prolonged QTc **(Choice C)**.

Q5. Identify malfunctioning PPM; failure to capture

Answer: C

This patient has had episodes of presyncope in the context of a malfunctioning pacemaker. Specifically, the ECG shows sinus rhythm with intermittent failure to capture. This patient has an atrial-sensing, ventricle-pacing PPM. Some pacing spikes on this ECG are not associated with a QRS. Furthermore, there are some QRS complexes that are not preceded by a pacing spike; these may represent either PVCs or native QRS complexes. The patient's PPM should be interrogated to determine the type of malfunction occurring with the device, and a lead revision should be performed inpatiently **(Choice C)**.

Q6. Identify 2nd degree AVB, Type I; recognize complications of Lyme disease

Answer: D

This patient has a clinical history concerning for Lyme carditis. The ECG demonstrates normal sinus rhythm with 2nd degree atrioventricular block, Mobitz Type I (Wenckebach). There is progressive PR segment lengthening of consecutive beats, followed by a "dropped" QRS complex. The QRS complex itself is likely to be narrow (<120 ms in duration), as the block occurs at the level of the AV node. Due to the patient's 2nd degree AV block and symptoms, treatment with IV ceftriaxone is indicated **(Choice D)**.

Q7. Identify findings of pericarditis; integrate differential diagnosis and ECG findings

Answer: D

This patient's ECG demonstrates normal sinus rhythm but also has the hallmarks of acute pericarditis. There are diffuse, upwardly concave, >2 mm STE within the anterior (V1–V4), inferior (II, III, and aVF), and lateral (I, aVL) leads, along with associated PR depressions. A highly specific finding for pericarditis is a PR elevation in Lead aVR, also shown in this ECG. In contrast to a STEMI, there are no reciprocal ST depressions present, and the STEs occur in multiple vascular territories. The mainstay of therapy for (viral) pericarditis is NSAIDs and colchicine **(Choice D)**.

Q8. Identify left ventricular hypertrophy; recognize ECG signs of structural heart disease

Answer: E

The patient in this vignette likely has hypertension, with classic features on her ECG. Although sex and age play a role in the calculation, the following criteria are useful in this case: By Sokolow–Lyon criteria, the S-wave in V1 plus the R-wave in V5 (or V6, whichever is taller) is >35 mm. By Cornell criteria, the R-wave in aVL is >11 mm (not present in this tracing). There are secondary repolarization abnormalities along leads V5 and V6, as there are discordant ST depressions with T-wave inversions—likely a consequence of hypertension. Technically, cardiac imaging (such as with an echocardiogram) is required to diagnose LVH. In order to diagnose hypertension, ambulatory BP monitoring is the next step **(Choice E)**.

Q9. Identify prior infarct; localization of myocardial infarction

Answer: B

This patient has suffered a myocardial infarction, as there are ST-segment elevations in Leads II, III, and aVF with reciprocal changes in the anterior and lateral leads. This is indicative of a STEMI; the absence of pathological Q-waves despite the presence of ST-segment elevations is indicative of an acute MI. Q-wave formation on ECG after an acute MI is indicative of myocardial scarring. An infarction pattern along the inferior leads implicates the right coronary artery as the culprit in most cases **(Choice B)**.

Q10. Identify typical findings in hyperkalemia; appropriate treatment

Answer: C

ECG of patient with hyperkalemia may show peaked T-waves, a widened QRS complex (>120 ms in duration), and a prolonged QTc (>500 ms). If untreated, hyperkalemia can induce fatal arrhythmias. As hyperkalemia worsens, ECGs will lose discernable P-waves and adopt a sinusoidal morphology, as seen here. While initial treatment to lower elevated serum potassium levels is warranted, IV calcium should be considered whenever ECG changes are present to stabilize the myocardium **(Choice C)**.

Q11. Identify atrial fibrillation; indications for anticoagulation

Answer: A

The patient has a physical exam and ECG that is indicative of atrial fibrillation. The ECG lacks discernable P-waves, instead showing "f" waves of inconsistent voltage, duration, morphology, and frequency, often with an atrial rate in excess of 500 BPM. The RR interval is irregularly irregular, and no clear pattern is evident. Atrial activity is best observed in the proximal precordial leads (V1 and V2) but may also be seen in the inferior leads (II, III, and aVF). Due to her elevated risk of thromboembolic stroke and CHA_2DS_2VASc score, the patient should be started on anticoagulation **(Choice A)**.

Q12. Identify CHB; indications for transvenous pacing and PPM

Answer: B

This patient has presented with syncope that is cardiogenic in etiology. His ECG reveals 3rd degree AV block, also known as complete heart block. Atrial and ventricular activity is dissociated from one another, leading to separate atrial and ventricular rhythms. No QRS complexes are "dropped" in CHB, but there may be retrograde P-waves buried within the QRS complex or T-waves. The PP interval and RR interval remain constant. Syncope from CHB requires temporary pacing until a permanent pacemaker can be inserted **(Choice B)**.

Q13. Identify incomplete RBBB in an asymptomatic patient

Answer: A

The patient has no cardiac complaints but does have an incomplete RBBB on his ECG. Like a complete RBBB, an incomplete RBBB will have an rSR' morphology in Lead

V1 and V2. However, a complete RBBB will have a QRS duration >120 ms, whereas an incomplete RBBB will have a QRS duration of 90–120 ms. An incomplete RBBB is a normal variant in some healthy adults but may also be due to chest wall deformities, RVH, and other cardiovascular conditions. In the absence of cardiac symptoms, no further work-up is required **(Choice A)**.

Q14. Normal Sinus Rhythm; indications for cardiac event monitoring in cryptogenic stroke

Answer: B

This patient has had multiple, small strokes that may be embolic in mechanism. The ECG demonstrates sinus rhythm, but this does not rule out the possibility of occult atrial fibrillation (or atrial flutter) that could have caused a cardioembolic stroke. In the absence of other clear etiologies, an implantable loop recorder could be considered to rule out paroxysmal arrhythmias that could have contributed to the patient's presentation **(Choice B)**.

Q15. Sinus Bradycardia; recognizing physiological sinus bradycardia in athletes and healthy patients

Answer: E

This patient has had chest wall trauma due to a mechanical fall. His exam and CT scan are pointing toward a musculoskeletal pathology. His ECG reveals sinus bradycardia but otherwise lacks ST changes, pathological Q-waves, and other signs of ischemia. Due to his cardiovascular exercise regimen, he has likely developed a physiological sinus bradycardia from increased vagal tone. The patient has no concerning pathology, so he may resume training when he feels ready **(Choice E)**.

Q16. Sinus Tachycardia; not beta-blocking sinus tachycardia/knowing causes of sinus tachycardia

Answer: B

The patient has developed diverticulitis associated with a fever, leading to pain (as well as stimulating his underlying anxiety). His ECG demonstrates sinus tachycardia without concomitant ST changes or other signs of ischemia. In the context of infection/inflammation, pain, fever, hypovolemia, and anxiety (from a catecholamine surge), sinus tachycardia may be appropriate. In the context of the above, sinus tachycardia should not be blunted with beta-blockers **(Choice B)**.

Q17. J-point elevation: Identify non-pathological early repolarization in a young, healthy patient

Answer: C

This young patient without any cardiac history is concerned about "ST changes" seen on a previous ECG. His current ECG reveals J-point elevation (a "take-off" at the beginning of the ST segment) along the precordial leads with a notching of the R-wave. This phenomenon is most commonly seen along Leads V1–V4, as is the case in this tracing. Of note, J-point elevation (also known as early repolarization) does not have reciprocal ST depressions. In an asymptomatic patient, no work-up is necessary, and reassurance should be provided **(Choice C)**.

Q18. LAA; identify rheumatic fever as a precursor to mitral stenosis, and the possibility of producing P-mitrale

Answer: A

This patient has mitral stenosis, likely from rheumatic heart disease stemming from an infection during her childhood. She has characteristic ECG changes associated with mitral stenosis. Her EKG shows a notched P-wave >120 ms in duration, also known as "P mitrale." The P-wave in V1 has a pronounced negative tail >1 mm deep, which is also consistent with LAA and can be seen with mitral stenosis **(Choice A)**.

Q19. Ectopic Atrial Rhythm: Identify ectopic atrial foci, even when the patient is being ventricularly paced

Answer: D

The patient's pre-cardioversion ECG demonstrates atrial. His post-cardioversion tracing shows a regular rhythm with 1:1 conduction between the atria (P-wave) and ventricles (QRS complex), but the P-wave axis is abnormal. Sinus rhythm is defined as positive (upright) P-waves in the inferior leads (II, III, and aVF), with a biphasic P-wave in Lead V1. This ECG shows negative P-wave deflections in the inferior leads, implying another atrial focus different from the SA node has overdrive-suppressed the sinus node. This ECG demonstrates an ectopic atrial rhythm with a normally-functioning ventricular pacemaker, as evidenced by pacer spikes at the beginning of each QRS complex **(Choice D)**.

Q20. 2nd Degree AV Block, Type I (Wenkebach); display knowledge of the management of this asymptomatic rhythm

Answer: E

This patient has developed 2nd degree AV block Mobitz Type I (Wenckebach) at some point after he received his cardioversion. The ECG demonstrates progressively increasing PR segments until a beat is dropped (non-conducted), although the periodicity of Mobitz Type I AV block may be difficult to ascertain if concomitant sinus arrhythmia is present. In an asymptomatic patient, this rhythm requires no specific treatment, and reassurance should be provided **(Choice E).**

Q21. 2nd Degree AV Block, Type II; indication to implant a PPM due to advanced conduction system disease

Answer: B

The patient's ECG and telemetry are indicative of 2nd degree AV block Mobitz Type II, which is a pathological finding on ECG. This is evident from the fact that the PR interval remains constant, but a QRS complex is "dropped" anyway. Irrespective of symptoms, this degree of conduction system disease needs to be treated with permanent pacing **(Choice B).**

Q22. Complete heart block; indications for transvenous pacing and PPM placement

Answer: B

The patient in this vignette has an ECG tracing that shows 3rd degree atrioventricular block, also known as "complete" heart block. The atria and ventricles beat independently of each other, typically with the atrial rate being faster than the ventricular rate.

The ventricular rate is mediated by a focus in the AV junction or distally in the conducting system. In a patient with syncope from CHB, a temporary pacing wire is indicated urgently if pacemaker implantation cannot be performed immediately **(Choice B).**

Q23. Multifocal Atrial Tachycardia: Identify MAT in a COPD exacerbation, and give supportive care for the underlying trigger

Answer: C

The patient developed an atrial tachyarrhythmia in the context of acute or chronic COPD. This tracing demonstrates at least three distinct P-wave morphologies with varying PP and PR intervals. This is consistent with multifocal atrial tachycardia, a condition usually arising in the context of pulmonary conditions (such as COPD exacerbations) causing atrial ectopy. Hypoxemia leads to multiple atrial foci depolarizing, which explains the different P-wave morphologies from one beat to the next. Treating the underlying medical condition is the most appropriate management **(Choice C)**.

Q24. Atrial fibrillation with CVR; indications for antiplatelet and anticoagulation by using the CHA2DS2VASc score

Answer: E

The ECG tracing in this patient reveals atrial fibrillation with a controlled ventricular response—the term "controlled" is used because the HR is between 60–100 BPM. The patient's arrhythmia was likely a consequence of "holiday heart," in which atrial fibrillation is brought on by alcohol use. The CHA_2DS_2VASc score estimates stroke risk in patients with atrial fibrillation, even in patients who convert back to sinus rhythm. This patient has a score of 0, so no antiplatelet or anticoagulation regimen is required in the long term **(Choice E)**.

Q25. Atrial Fibrillation with RVR; contraindications to using rhythm control without anticoagulation or TEE/CTCA

Answer: C

This patient's ECG demonstrates atrial fibrillation with a rapid ventricular response. Classic hallmarks of atrial fibrillation, such as f-waves and the lack of an isoelectric baseline, are present. "Rapid ventricular response" refers to the fact that the ventricular rate is >100 BPM. Rate control strategies, including metoprolol, diltiazem, and digoxin, are all appropriate. Electrolyte derangements, such as hypomagnesemia, can contribute to this arrhythmia. Rhythm control (amiodarone) should not be attempted in the absence of anticoagulation, especially if left atrial appendage thrombus has not been ruled out **(Choice C)**.

Q26. Atrial flutter: Identify important attributes of atrial flutter, in contrast to atrial fibrillation

Answer: C

The ECG for this patient is indicative of atrial flutter. The atrial rate in atrial flutter is typically between 240–340 BPM, with F-waves that are classically described as having a "sawtooth" morphology. Like atrial fibrillation, Lead V1 may have discrete deflections, in contrast to the flutter waves present in other leads. The ratio of F-waves to QRS complexes is usually an even number (such as 2:1), with conduction ratios of 1:1 and 3:1 being less common. The cavo-tricuspid isthmus is the site of typical atrial flutter, as is the case here **(Choice C)**.

Q27. AIVR: Identify the clinical significance of AIVR (reperfusion) after cardiac catheterization

Answer: A

This ECG demonstrates an accelerated idioventricular rhythm (AIVR). The reverse R-wave progression and Northwestern axis are due to the patient's history of dextrocardia. The term "accelerated" refers to a rate between 60–110 BPM. The rhythm is usually regular, with a QRS that has a similar morphology to that of premature ventricular contraction (PVC). There exists competition between the sinus node and an ectopic focus from a ventricle, which produces fusion beats and AV dissociation. AIVR often indicates reperfusion of a previously occluded coronary artery and may be seen after a successful percutaneous coronary intervention **(Choice A)**.

Q28. Torsades de pointes: Identify the consequences of using multiple QTc-prolonger medications, and management of TdP

Answer: D

This patient's telemetry strip shows that he developed torsades de pointes (TdP, "twisting of the points"). TdP is characterized by an antecedent prolonged QT interval that progresses to irregular episodes of ventricular tachyarrhythmias. The ventricular rate is between 200–280 BPM, with a wide-QRS morphology >120 ms that may resemble a sine wave. The QRS complexes alternate in terms of deflection and amplitude. TdP is treated with magnesium infusions and unsynchronized cardioversion if the patient becomes pulseless **(Choice D)**.

Q29. Supraventricular Tachycardia; delineate SVT from VT using the Brugada criteria

Answer: B

The ECG in this vignette shows supraventricular tachycardia with aberrancy. In patients with VT, the RR interval is typically regular and may be associated with AV dissociation. Fusion complexes and capture complexes may also be seen with ventricular tachycardia. The Brugada criteria is used to delineate SVT with aberrancy from VT; parameters like the R-to-S nadir being >100 ms and morphological criteria for atypical bundle branch blocks in Leads V1 and V6 favor VT when present **(Choice B)**.

Q30. MMVT; recall management for dealing with VT with or without a pulse

Answer: E

This patient developed monomorphic ventricular tachycardia with a pulse, complicated by altered mental status. The ECG shows a wide QRS rhythm that rules in for VT, based upon the Brugada and aVR criteria algorithms. Amiodarone should be given for shockable rhythms in stable patients, while defibrillation should be used in patients in cardiac arrest from VT **(Choice E)**.

BIBLIOGRAPHY

1. AbdElkareem, T. S., Ahmed, T. A., & Mohamed, L. A. (2023, April). *Left atrial remodeling in patients with severe rheumatic mitral stenosis and sinus rhythm using two-dimensional and three-dimensional speckle tracking echocardiography.* Cardiology Research. https://www.ncbi.nlm.nih.gov/pmc/articles/PMC10116933/
2. Brugada, P., Brugada, J., Mont, L., Smeets, J., & Andries, E. W. (1991, May 1). *A new approach to the differential diagnosis of a regular tachycardia with a wide QRS complex.* Circulation. https://pubmed.ncbi.nlm.nih.gov/2022022/
3. Buelt, A., Richards, A., & Jones, A. L. (2021, June 15). *Hypertension: New guidelines from the International Society of Hypertension.* American Family Physician. https://www.aafp.org/pubs/afp/issues/2021/0615/p763.html
4. Chow, B. J. W., Cheung, M., Prosperi-Porta, G., Tavoosi, A., Motazedian, P., Guler, E. C., Yam, Y., Burwash, I., Dennie, C., & Golian, M. (2024, June 17). *Left atrial imaging prior to cardioversion: Leveraging …* JACC: Cardiovascular Imaging. https://www.jacc.org/doi/10.1016/j.jcmg.2023.12.009
5. De Jong, A. M., Maass, A. H., Oberdorf-Maass, S. U., Van Veldhuisen, D. J., Van Gilst, W. H., & Van Gelder, I. C. (2010, November 11). *Mechanisms of atrial structural changes caused by stretch occurring before and during early atrial fibrillation.* OUP Academic. https://academic.oup.com/cardiovascres/article/89/4/754/261018
6. Indraratna, P., Tardo, D., Delves, M., Szirt, R., & Ng, B. (2020, March). *Measurement and management of QT interval prolongation for general physicians.* Journal of General Internal Medicine. https://www.ncbi.nlm.nih.gov/pmc/articles/PMC7080915/
7. Ismail, T. F. (2020, January). *Acute pericarditis: Update on diagnosis and management.* Clinical Medicine (London, England). https://www.ncbi.nlm.nih.gov/pmc/articles/PMC6964178/
8. Jowett, N. I., Thompson, D. R., & Pohl, J. E. F. (1989, April 1). *Temporary transvenous cardiac pacing: 6 years experience in one Coronary Care Unit.* OUP Academic. https://academic.oup.com/pmj/article/65/762/211/7044313
9. Kadish, A. H., Buxton, A. E., Kennedy, H. L., Knight, B. P., Mason, J. W., Schuger, C. D., Tracy, C. M., Winters, W. L., Boone, A. W., Elnicki, M., Hirshfeld, J. W., Lorell, B. H., Rodgers, G. P., Tracy, C. M., & Weitz, H. H. (2001). *ACC/AHA clinical competence statement on electrocardiography and ambulatory electrocardiography. Circulation, 104*(25), 3169–3178. https://doi.org/10.1161/circ.104.25.3169
10. Kusumoto, F. M., Schoenfeld, M. H., Barrett, C., Edgerton, J. R., Ellenbogen, K. A., Gold, M. R., Goldschlager, N. F., Hamilton, R. M., Joglar, J. A., Kim, R. J., Lee, R., Marine, J. E., McLeod, C. J., Oken, K. R., Patton, K. K., Pellegrini, C. N., Selzman, K. A., Thompson, A., & Varosy, P. D. (2018, November 6). *2018 ACC/AHA/HRS guideline on the evaluation and management of patients with bradycardia and cardiac conduction delay: Executive summary: A report of the American College of Cardiology/American Heart Association Task Force on Clinical Practice Guidelines, and the Heart Rhythm Society | Circulation.* Circulation. https://www.ahajournals.org/doi/10.1161/CIR.0000000000000627
11. Lane, D. A., & Lip, G. Y. H. (2012, August 14). *Use of the CHA2DS2-vasc and has-bled scores to aid decision making for thromboprophylaxis in nonvalvular atrial fibrillation | circulation.* Circulation. https://www.ahajournals.org/doi/10.1161/CIRCULATIONAHA.111.060061
12. Moya, A., Sutton, R., Ammirati, F., Blanc, J.-J., Brignole, M., Dahm, J. B., Deharo, J.-C., Gajek, J., Gjesdal, K., Krahn, A., Massin, M., Pepi, M., Pezawas, T., Ruiz Granell, R., Sarasin, F., Ungar, A., van Dijk, J. G., Walma, E. P., & Wieling, W. (2009, November).

Guidelines for the diagnosis and management of syncope (version 2009). European Heart Journal. https://www.ncbi.nlm.nih.gov/pmc/articles/PMC3295536/

13. Mushiyakh, Y., Dangaria, H., Qavi, S., Ali, N., Pannone, J., & Tompkins, D. (2012, January 26). *Treatment and pathogenesis of acute hyperkalemia.* Journal of Community Hospital Internal Medicine Perspectives. https://www.ncbi.nlm.nih.gov/pmc/articles/PMC3714047/
14. O'Gara, P. T., Kushner, F. G., Ascheim, D. D., Casey, D. E., Chung, M. K., de Lemos, J. A., Ettinger, S. M., Fang, J. C., Fesmire, F. M., Franklin, B. A., Granger, C. B., Krumholz, H. M., Linderbaum, J. A., Morrow, D. A., Newby, L. K., Ornato, J. P., Ou, N., Radford, M. J., Tamis-Holland, J. E., ... Zhao, D. X. (2012, December 17). *ACC/AHA guidelines for the management of patients with ST-elevation myocardial infarction—executive summary | circulation.* Circulation. https://www.ahajournals.org/doi/full/10.1161/01.cir.0000134791.68010.fa
15. O'Keefe, J. H., Pogwizd, S. M., Freed, M. S., & Hammill, S. C. (2015). *The ECG Criteria Book* (2nd ed.). Jones & Bartlett Learning.
16. PérezRodon, J., FranciscoPascual, J., RivasGándara, N., RocaLuque, I., Bellera, N., & MoyaMitjans, À. (2014, December 31). *Cryptogenic stroke and role of Loop Recorder.* Journal of Atrial Fibrillation. https://www.ncbi.nlm.nih.gov/pmc/articles/PMC5135209/
17. Perman, S. H., Elmer, J., Maciel, C. B., Uzendu, A., May, T., Mumma, B. E., Bartos, J. A., Rodriguez, A. J., Kurz, M. C., Panchal, A. R., & Rittenberger, J. C. (2023, December 18). *2023 American Heart Association focused update on ...* Circulation. https://www.ahajournals.org/doi/10.1161/CIR.0000000000001194
18. Phillips, J., Hazard, P., Berlinerblau, R., Levine, J., Iseri, L., Higbee, M., Marchlinski, F., Arsura, E., Strickberger, S., Zeevi, B., Byrd, R., Bourdillon, P., Shine, K., Wang, K., Lipson, M., Kones, R., Scher, D., Habibzadeh, M., Parillo, J., ... Rall, T. (2004, February 19). *Multifocal atrial tachycardia: Mechanisms, clinical correlates, and treatment.* American Heart Journal. https://www.sciencedirect.com/science/article/abs/pii/0002870389902755
19. Sabbagh, E., Abdelfattah, T., Karim, M. M., Farah, A., Grubb, B., & Karim, S. (2020, February 15). *Causes of failure to capture in pacemakers and implantable cardioverter-defibrillators.* The Journal of Innovations in Cardiac Rhythm Management. https://www.ncbi.nlm.nih.gov/pmc/articles/PMC7192127/
20. Shu, J., Gussak, I., Francis, J., Potet, F., & Kalla, H. (2006, March 30). *Early repolarization syndrome: Is it always benign?* International Journal of Cardiology. https://www.sciencedirect.com/science/article/abs/pii/S0167527306001100
21. Thomas, S. H. L., & Behr, E. R. (2015, October 26). *Pharmacological treatment of acquired QT prolongation and Torsades de Pointes.* British Journal of Clinical Pharmacology. https://pubmed.ncbi.nlm.nih.gov/26183037/
22. Turkelsen, C. J., Sorensen, J. T., Kaltoft, A. K., Nielsen, S. S., Thuesen, L., Botker, H.-E., & Lassen, J. F. (2009, December 15). *Prevalence and significance of accelerated idioventricular rhythm in patients with ST-elevation myocardial infarction treated with primary percutaneous coronary intervention.* The American Journal of Cardiology. https://pubmed.ncbi.nlm.nih.gov/19962468/
23. Vereckei, A. (2014, August). *Current algorithms for the diagnosis of wide QRS complex tachycardias.* Current Cardiology Reviews. https://www.ncbi.nlm.nih.gov/pmc/articles/PMC4040878/
24. Wellens, H. J. (2009, November 1). *The ECG in localizing the culprit lesion in acute inferior myocardial infarction: A plea for lead V4R?* OUP Academic. https://academic.oup.com/europace/article/11/11/1421/444266

Index

Note: *Italic* page numbers refer to *figures*.

R

S

T

V

W